Songs You Know By Heart
A Simple Guide for Using Music in Dementia Care

When words fail, music speaks.

Mary Sue Wilkinson

© 2016 by Mary Sue Wilkinson

Published by Mission Point Press
Traverse City, Michigan

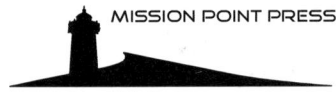

ISBN: 978-1-943995-02-8

Library of Congress Control Number: 2016901578

All rights reserved. No part of this book may be reproduced or transmitted in any form or by any means, electronic or mechanical, including photocopying, recording or by any information storage and retrieval system with the exception of a reviewer who may quote brief passages without the written permission from the author. For information, contact: Mary Sue Wilkinson, Singing Heart to Heart, 4169 Summerhill Road, Traverse City, MI 49684; 231-233-2948, www.SingingHeartToHeart.com.

Cover Photo: Pauline Weaner with Mary Sue Wilkinson, Photography by Myrna Jacobs.

Interior Photos: Photography by Myrna Jacobs, Mary Sue Wilkinson, Ann Ballou, Janine Andrew and other family members.

All photos used by permission.

Cover Design: George Foster, Foster Covers
www.fostercovers.com

Interior Design: Mission Point Press
www.missionpointpress.com

PLEASE NOTE: QUANTITY DISCOUNTS ARE AVAILABLE TO YOUR COMPANY, NON-PROFIT OR EDUCATIONAL INSTITUTION for reselling, educational purposes, training, or gifts. For more information please contact Singing Heart to Heart, 4169 Summerhill Road, Traverse City, MI 49684, 231-233-2948, marysue@singinghearttoheart.com.

www.SingingHeartToHeart.com

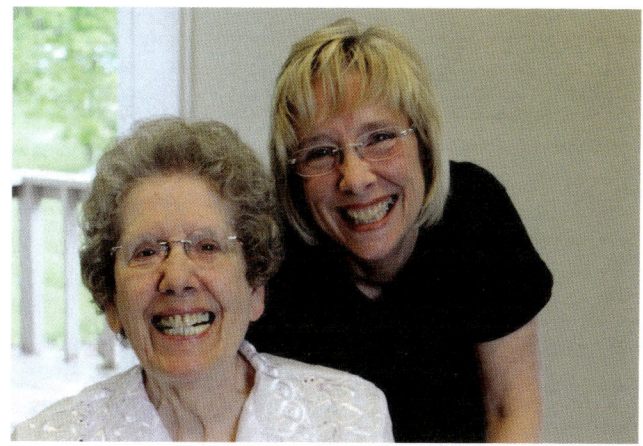

This book is dedicated with love to the memory of Polly Ballou.

Polly lived with Alzheimer's for many years but never lost her smile or her loving heart. First and foremost a mom, Polly raised her children with love and kindness and a steadfast faith, alongside her beloved husband Ken. Polly's talents and generosity touched the lives of many in her community, her church, her neighborhood, her kindergarten classroom, and within her extended family. Through music and the loving care of her devoted daughter Ann, Polly was able to experience joy and continue to express love, even when words failed her.

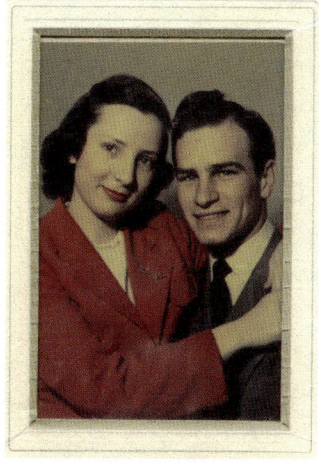

This book is also dedicated to the memory of my mother, Marilyn Wilkinson, who taught me to sing. A greater gift I have never received. And to my father, John Wilkinson, who taught me to dance and whose love holds me steady every day.

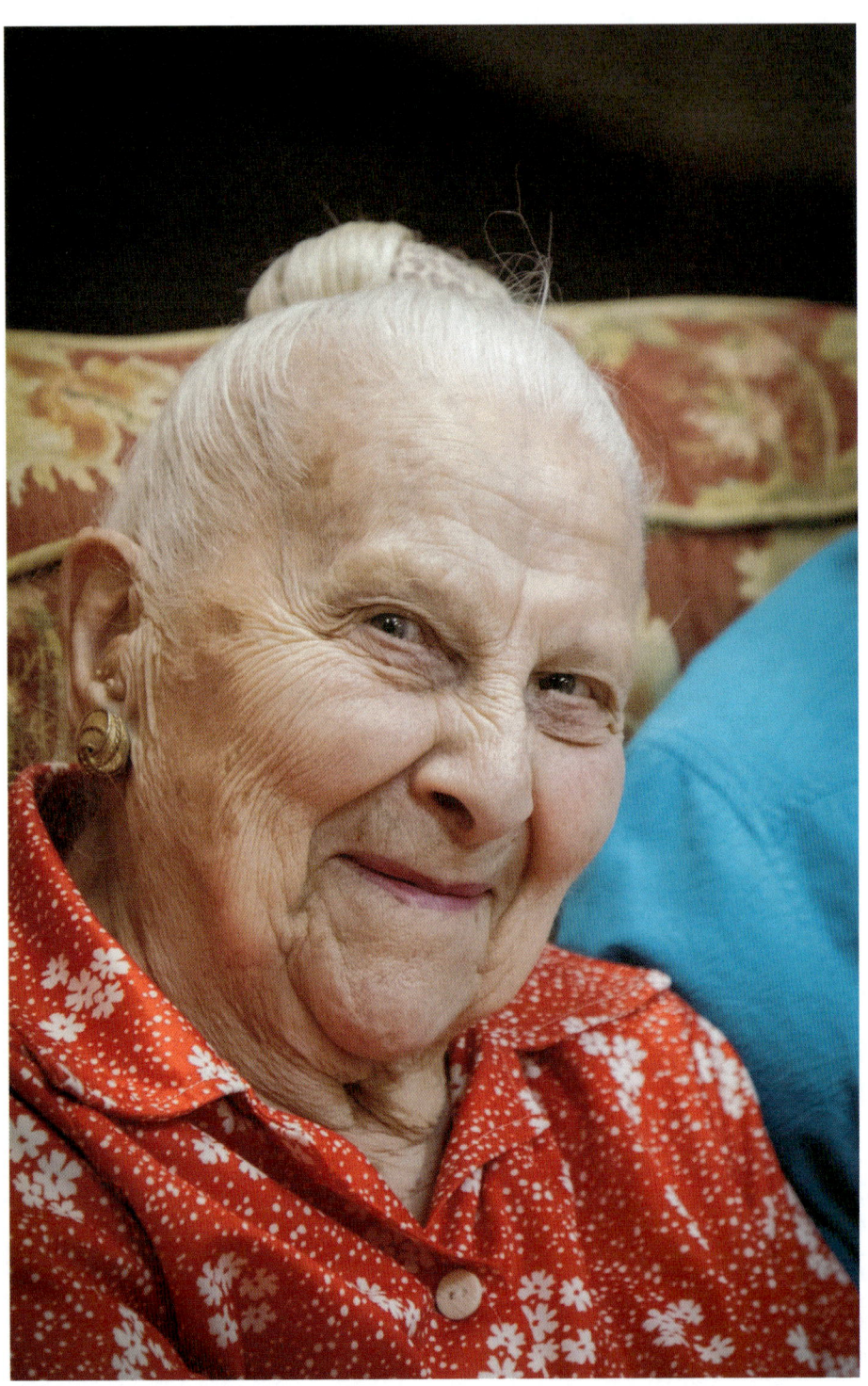

Contents

Foreword ...... *vi*

A Note from the Author ...... *ix*

Introduction ...... *xi*

Chapter 1: How and Why Music Improves Quality of Life *1*
(Benefits We All Enjoy Through Music; Benefits for the Caregiver, Family Member, and Activity Director; Benefits During Hospice Care)

Chapter 2: Let's Get Started: A Basic Overview *7*
(Six Key Steps for Success; Tips and Tricks to Keep in Your Toolbox; What if…)

Chapter 3: Let's Sing! *13*
(Ready, Set, Sing!; Choosing Songs; List of Six Simple Songs; Two Songs to Keep in Your Back Pocket)

Chapter 4: Let's Move to Music! *19*
(Ready, Set, Move!; List of Movement Suggestions; A 15 Minute Music and Movement Plan)

Chapter 5: Song by Song: Using the *Songs You Know By Heart* Recording *27*
(Directions for Downloading the Songs)

Chapter 6: Frequently Asked Questions *39*

Chapter 7: Introducing Teepa Snow's GEMS™ Dementia Classification Model *47*

Chapter 8: Connecting Music to the GEMS™ Stages of Dementia *57*

Online Resources *70*

Bibliography *71*

About Mary Sue Wilkinson and Singing Heart to Heart™ *72*

About Teepa Snow and Positive Approach to Care™ *73*

Foreword

Throughout my many years of providing support and care for people living with dementia and their families and care partners, I have found the power of music and rhythm to be one of the greatest gifts I can offer and accept in kind.

I love that more attention, awareness, and knowledge is being brought to bear on this generally retained skill. Yet there is still an absence of skill in applying what we know into daily habits and routines that make the most of what is possible, without overstressing the care provision system or misusing this gift and blessing.

Mary Sue Wilkinson's guide is just what is needed to move beyond using music as background noise, or simply putting headphones on people and letting them listen and enjoy songs in isolation. Using her suggestions and detailed recommendations truly offers ways to sustain or regain connections that we thought were lost or impossible—while respecting the individual's preferences and desires for alone time or engagement opportunities.

Using automatic social cues, patterns with music, and rhythmic movement to elicit responses can be life changing and love inducing. Music allows people to share what they feel, think, believe, and desire when they no longer can understand your questions or find the words.

Let me give you an example.

Although she had not spoken in three years, when a woman's husband sat in a chair next to her, she sweetly hummed "I Love You a Bushel and a Peck." Even so, her husband was distraught, telling me, "She never talks anymore. I'm not sure she even knows me."

"Oh, but I know she does," I replied. "Listen to the song she picked."

Realization crept over his face and he began to cry. "That was the song she used to sing to me after we had an argument," he said. So we sang the song together and I showed him how to "visually" offer his wife a hug, where she could see it. Then she looked directly into his eyes and mouthed, "I love you!"

What a gift to be part of that moment!

Enjoy what May Sue offers here, and use it well and wisely.

Teepa Snow

**Founder and President
of Positive Approach to Care™
www.teepasnow.com**

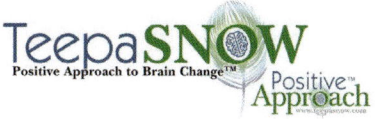

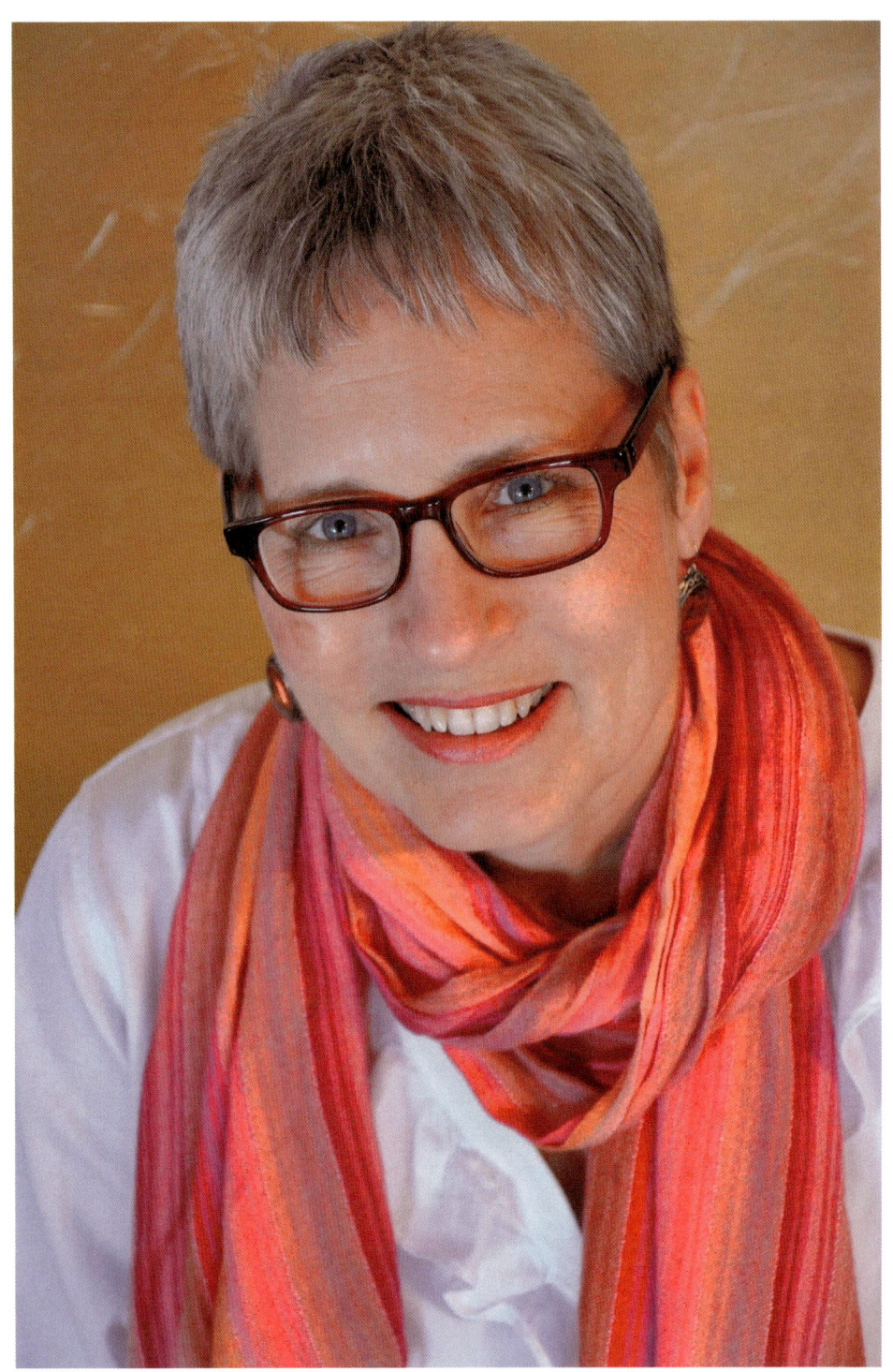

A Note From The Author

Whether you realize it or not, music has been accompanying you from your very first days, when your mother sang you a lullaby. Over the years music changed and you changed, too. But the songs of your youth are stored away in your brain, in their own special place. Hearing those songs allows you to access memories and feelings that may at other times seem too far away to enjoy. Science suggests that your brain is literally hardwired to connect music with memory.

I learned this from a very personal experience with my father-in-law, after he could no longer remember our names or carry on a conversation with us. He was a Church of the Brethren minister and when I sang the hymns he knew and loved, he was able to sing every word—and he even added harmony. It was an amazing transformation that clearly brought him joy. And more importantly, it gave us a way to stay connected.

Since then, I have spent hundreds of hours singing with older adults. Whether or not we have memory loss, music has the power to reach us and bring us happiness and connection. Music provides a unique opportunity to do something meaningful with others, no matter one's abilities or skills. With the **Songs You Know By Heart** recording and this guide, you, too, can harness the power of music. Drop me a line and let me know how it's going. I'd love to hear from you.

Mary Sue Wilkinson

**Founder and President of Singing Heart to Heart™
and the Young at Heart Music Program
www.SingingHeartToHeart.com**

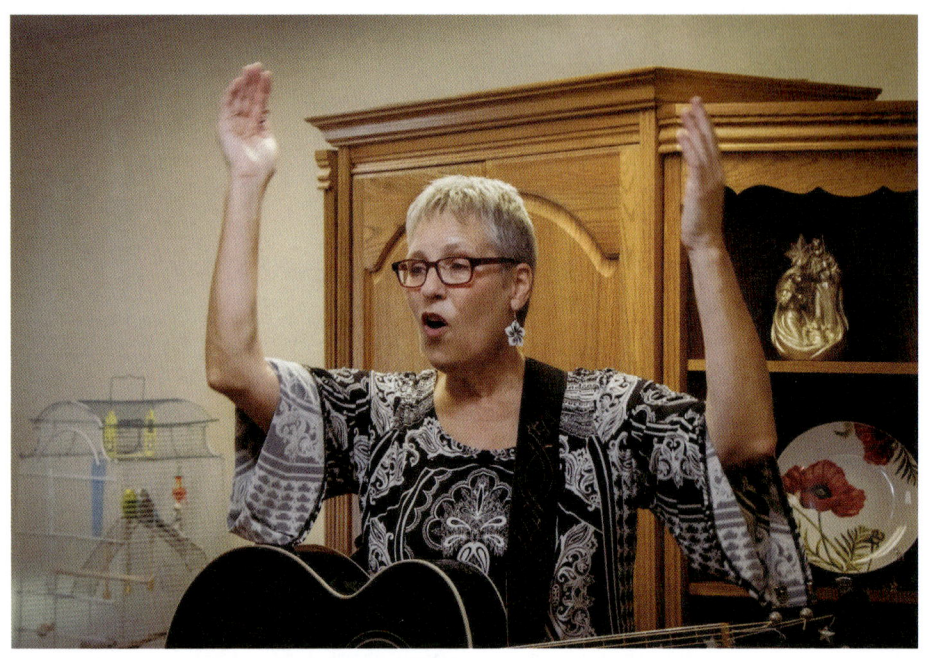
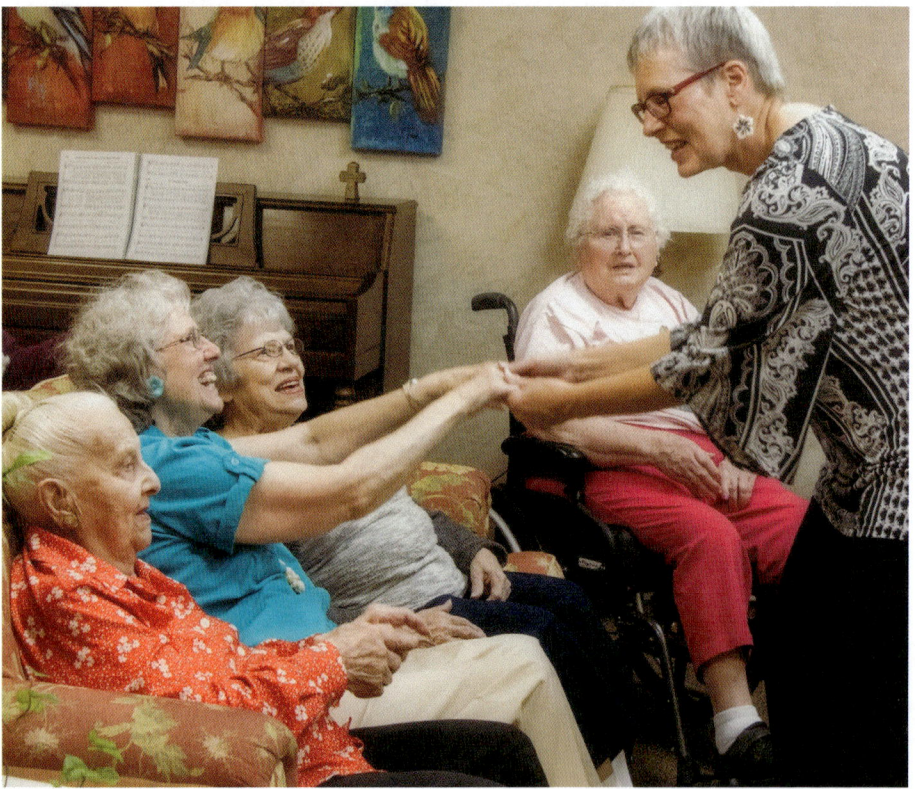

Introduction

- Do you interact with seniors or care for someone with dementia?

- Are you short on time and sometimes short on energy?

- Do you wish you could do something that would actually make your job easier?

- Are you looking for ways to focus on what people can do rather than on the support they need?

- Do you wish you had more tools to help the person you are caring for feel less restless, agitated and uncooperative—and more relaxed and happy?

- Do you wish you had a better (and easier) way to connect?

- Are you looking for a fun and meaningful activity that everyone can do together?

- Are you a music lover but not necessarily a musician?

- Would you like to have more music in your activity program but your budget is small?

Then this guide is for you.

Spend five minutes (yes, that's all the time it will take) to read about the many benefits of music. Then turn on the music and follow the simple directions for how to use the **Songs You Know By Heart** recording and other music.

Try one idea or try them all. The benefits to you and the person you care for are many. Rest assured that a little music goes a long way. Whether you are a caregiver, a family member, or an activity director, you are a very important person, uniquely qualified to help someone reap all the benefits and joy available through music.

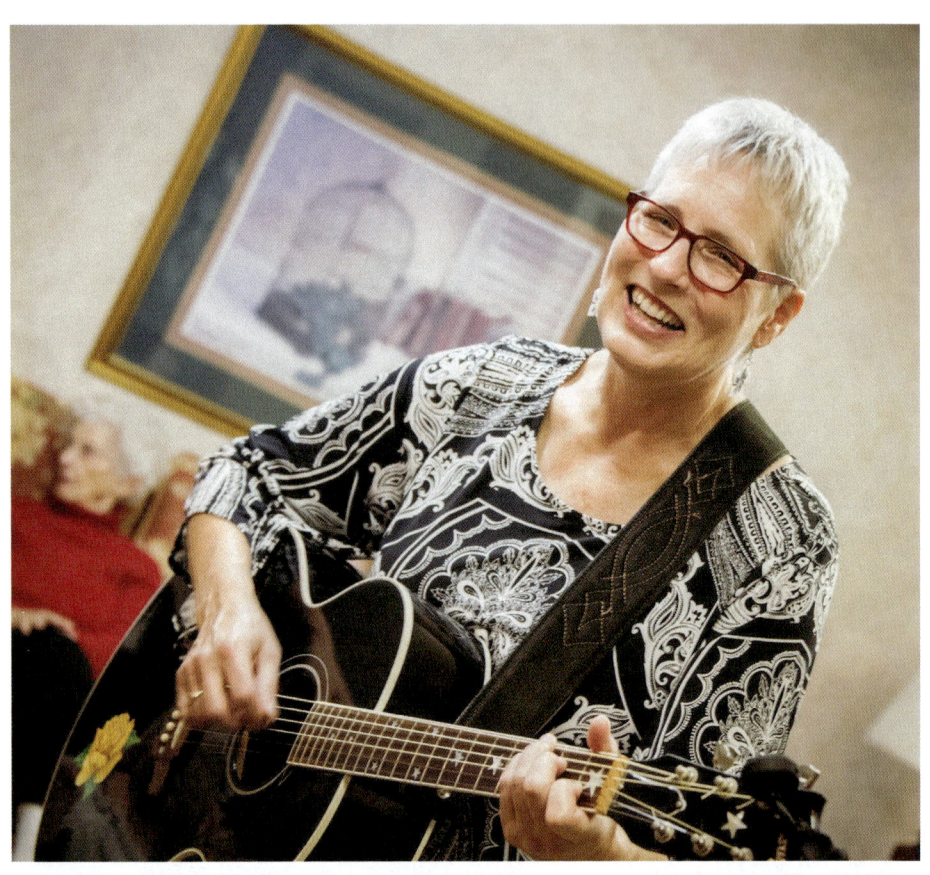
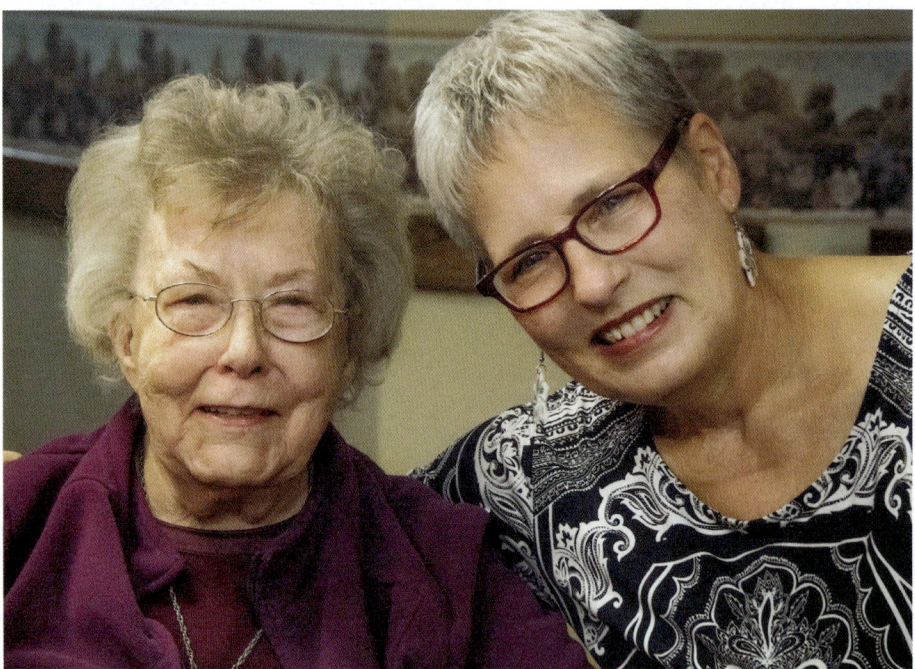

CHAPTER 1

How and Why Music Improves Quality of Life

Introduction

How is it that music improves the quality of life? Why does it matter? The answers are both complicated and simple.

The complicated part has to do with the brain, which science suggests is actually hardwired to connect music with memories. The songs of our youth are stored away in their own special spot in the brain. And no matter what happens, hearing those songs can allow us to access memories and feelings.

The simple part is that music affects how we feel. It stirs our souls. Have you ever heard a song on the radio that lifted your spirits or reminded you of someone or something you experienced? If so, you understand.

Most important to our purposes here, singing and music can simply make people happy. And happiness improves the quality of life for everyone.

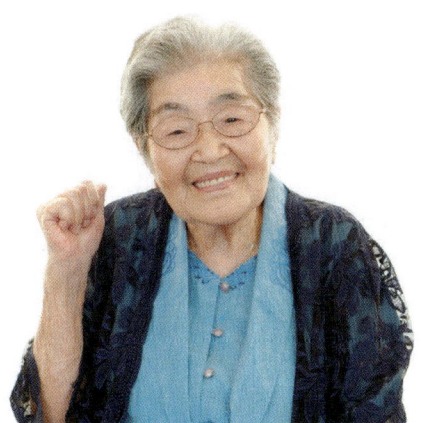

"Jean starts to live in the moment, and is carried away by the pure, simple joys of singing. I witness the feelings of inadequacy, anxiety, and fear dissipate as beautiful music comes out between you and Jean."

Kim Spencer, Caregiver

Benefits We All Enjoy Through Music

Singing together helps us connect. Singing together is a way we connect and maintain relationships even when other communication is difficult. Music is the soundtrack of our lives. It allows us to push back the silence and isolation. And everyone can sing. Really!

Singing together helps people feel like they belong. Singing together creates community and a sense of belonging. A music session can increase social interaction and communication, something those with dementia may not experience very often.

Singing helps people remember happy times. Music and singing awaken memory. Music is a pathway to emotional memories—familiar songs connect us with our history and our identities. Playing music from one's youth is the key. And don't miss the opportunity to talk about the memories that come up.

Singing familiar songs makes people feel comfortable and competent. People can often recall words to familiar songs from their youth, even when other memories are harder to access. As we age there are numerous ways that a person's world can shrink. Many older people don't drive, cook, go to work, or take care of their own house anymore. An activity that makes them feel competent is more important than you might think.

Music affects mood and lifts spirits. Before there was Prozac, there was music! Music can help ease depression and fear.

Music reaches everyone. Music can tap deep emotional memories, even for people living with severe memory loss. When we listen and sing, there is no right or wrong answer, no special skill needed, and no level of physical or mental ability required to engage with the music.

Singing gives people something fun to do together! Music and singing relieve boredom, one of the most difficult aspects of having dementia. People of all skill levels and all generations can successfully "do" music together and share a common and positive experience.

Music makes us want to move. Music gives people motivation to move and get some exercise. A sense of rhythm often remains even as other skills and abilities may change or decline.

Music is good for health. "A song a day keeps the doctor away" might indeed prove true. Research suggests that music can reduce anxiety and agitation; it can soothe or bring energy. It's good for your health!

Music helps people "live in the moment." Music sessions give people an opportunity to be present. They provide a break from the stress of living with dementia or other health concerns.

Music is comforting. People often have positive emotional recollections of their mother or father singing to them as young children. While they may not be able to recall those experiences, music can trigger the positive feelings associated with the memory.

Music Moment with Mary Sue

Barbara sits hunched over with her head tucked down so you can't see her eyes. But she is listening. Sometimes you can see her lips moving to the song. She is restless and often pushes herself up— with great effort— out of the chair or off the couch to wander across the room, often with one shoe off and one shoe on.

Today Barbara was wandering, and I asked her if she would like to dance with me. She nodded, and so I took her soft hands in mine and we moved together while I sang. She wore the faintest smile on her face as she moved her feet, side to side, dancing with me. When the dance was over, I thanked her, and she squeezed my hand.

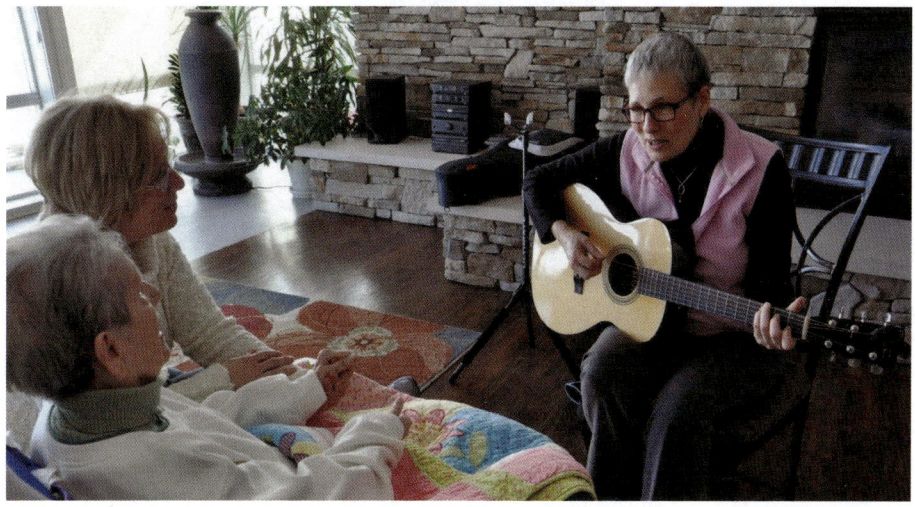

Benefits For The Caregiver, Family Member, and Activity Director

Music focuses on strengths rather than weaknesses. A music session can help staff and family focus on what older adults can *do* rather than on the daily support they need.

Music makes things easier. Let's face it: happy people are usually less difficult to care for. People who feel competent are likely to be less resistant to assistance in other areas of their lives. Bottom line, singing a simple song or playing music can literally make your job easier.

Music means fun. Music sessions are an opportunity to share a pleasurable and successful experience. Everyone can be involved because, in a way, it "levels the playing field."

Music builds relationships. Sharing a music session allows you to connect and have fun together which can strengthen and build relationships between staff, family members, and residents.

Music and dance bring tender connections. Dancing allows family members and spouses to experience a close emotional and physical connection with their loved one.

Music Moment with Mary Sue

Bob told me with a gentle smile, "I have memory loss." He was trying to recall the name of one of his favorite songs. Not knowing the song title didn't dampen his enthusiasm. As our music session began, he pushed up to his feet so that he could dance—often with his imaginary partner. He "held her" tenderly as he closed his eyes, wrapped his arms around himself, and caressed his own cheek. He swayed to the music and let the song take him to a place he remembered.

Bob likes rock and roll, Elvis, and "Blue Suede Shoes." He could be any man on any dance floor. He laughs as he dances. When we sing "Home on the Range," he joins me in adding the coyote's howls. Without being prompted, he adds the sound of a horn to "I've Been Working on the Railroad." He cups his hands around his mouth as we sing "Can't you hear the captain shouting, Dinah blow your horn!"

Bob's wife is visiting and tells me, "We both love music. We used to love to go out and dance all the time." I sing, "I'll be loving you, always…" and they dance.

Benefits During Hospice Care

Music is a time-out from talking. Often it's hard to know what to talk about when families are gathered in the hospice setting. Singing is something everyone can do to increase comfort and alleviate fears during a very difficult time.

Music is a pathway to meaning. Familiar songs may soothe when the unknown is looming. They can provide a pathway for reminiscing.

Music is a gift. Singing together is a way to actively do something for someone who is dying. It may comfort the singer as well as the hospice patient.

Music Moment with Mary Sue

Julie's hospital bed was set up in the living room. Surrounding her was the clutter of a life well lived. Several generations of family had gathered and crowded in to be with her during her last days. Little ones ran underfoot and young adult cousins stood around, at times awkward and at times jostling and joking, not sure how they were supposed to act. Julie's husband and friends were ever attentive, serving food and checking on her, offering comfort and conversation.

I arrived with my guitar and began to sing. Julie and her family called out their favorites: "You Are My Sunshine," then "Twinkle Little Star" for the toddlers. Secure now that it was ok to laugh and enjoy the moment, the cousins broke out an old rock and roll song. Spirits lifted with each song shared. Soon everyone was engaged in the music, together. Now everyone knew what to do. And it was ok to take a break from the grief.

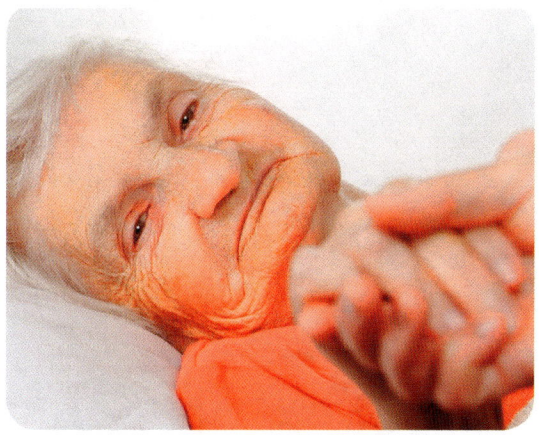

"Yesterday we visited my wife's Grandma, who just stopped chemo and doesn't have much longer. We sang Christmas carols for over an hour with her. It is amazing that when you don't have much left, you can still enjoy and co-create music."

Andy Evans, Grandson

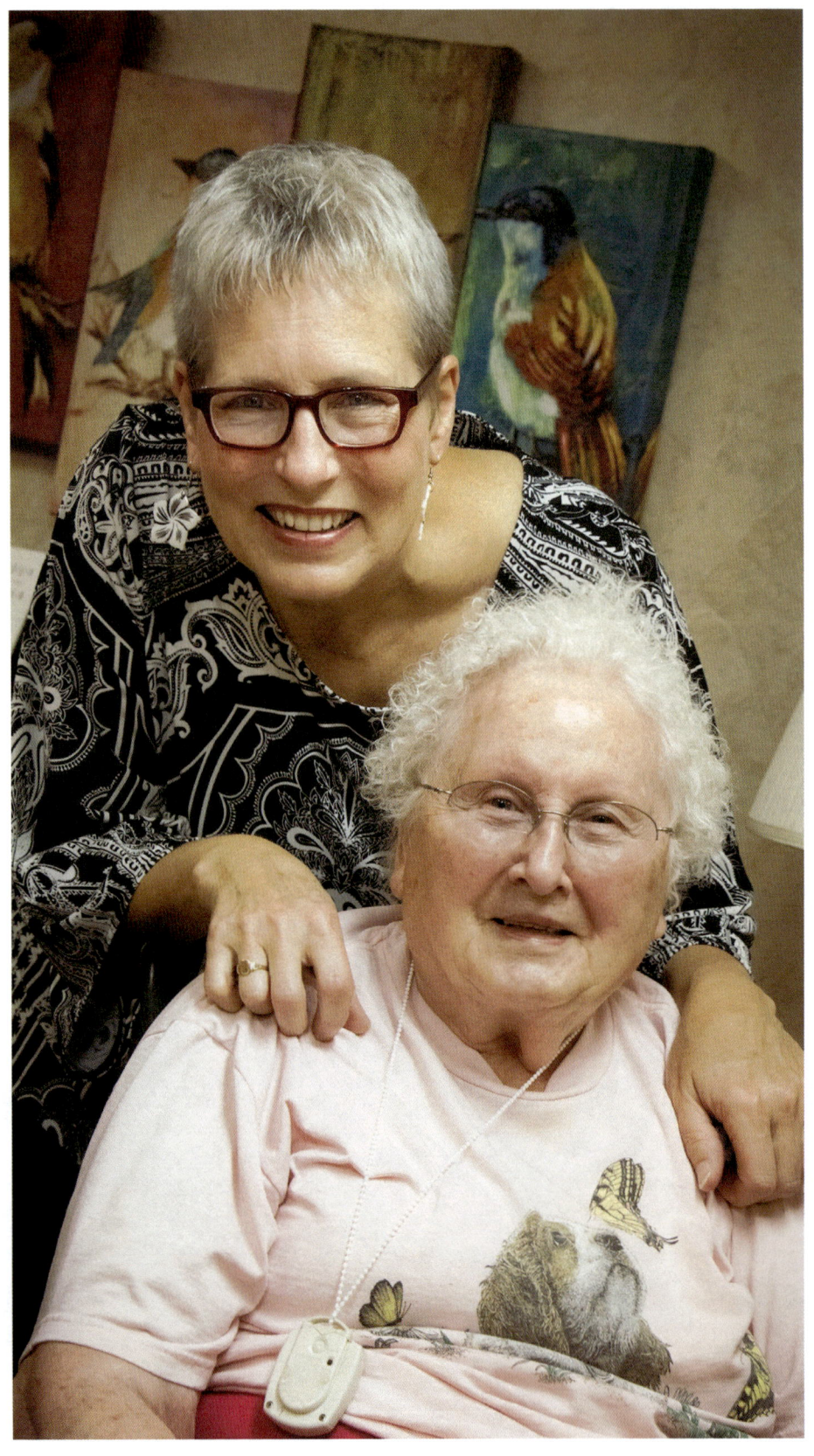

Chapter 2

Let's Get Started: A Basic Overview

Six key steps for success

Know your audience and respect who they are and what they need. Some may need and enjoy having you close by; others may prefer to be on the fringes watching.

Invite participation, but don't ask permission. Don't give folks a chance to say no! Instead, muster up your enthusiasm, a big smile, and some movement to get a better response when you announce, "It's time to sing!" Visual cues are the most effective way to reach people with dementia.

Help them begin. People with dementia often have a hard time getting started. If you notice someone not singing or joining in, your smiling presence nearby may help. But be respectful. Don't overwhelm them. Cue people visually. Our eyes are number one in terms of how we get information. For people with dementia, your words may have lost some or all meaning.

Use the "Simple 15-Minute Music and Movement Plan" provided in Chapter 4 to get you going. Then develop your own playlists as you explore the rest of the *Songs You Know By Heart* recording.

Wind down. Mark the end of music time with a closing song, such as "When You're Smiling" or "Goodnight Ladies."

Keep track. You will learn which songs are the favorites. Repeat those often. Keep notes and jot down your plans using the pages provided in the back of this guide.

Tips & Tricks to Keep in Your Toolbox

- **Be a cheerleader.** Your enthusiasm will be contagious. Keep up the encouragement. Things might begin slowly, so don't give up too soon.

- **Get to know which songs they like.** Songs from their childhood and youth are most important. Find out which songs on the recording they like. Then ask questions of anyone who can provide information, so you can expand your repertoire. Personal preferences matter.

- **Observe**. Keep your eyes open and look closely. Pay attention to facial expressions. Are toes tapping, fingers moving? Do people look comfortable? Are they participating? Responses may be very small and may take time to show up. Be a good detective.

- **Repetition is rewarding.** Don't be afraid to keep repeating songs and activities. This allows slower-moving brains to catch up.

- **On cue.** Consider using one song over and over as a cue. It could be a good morning song, a good night song, a hello song, a time-to-get-dressed song, or a song for bathing.

- **Mix it up.** Make your own playlist. You don't have to follow the order of the *Songs You Know By Heart* recording.

"I played your CD for Kathy today and she loved it. It was the most relaxed I have seen her in a long time."

Merri Rose, Daughter-in-law

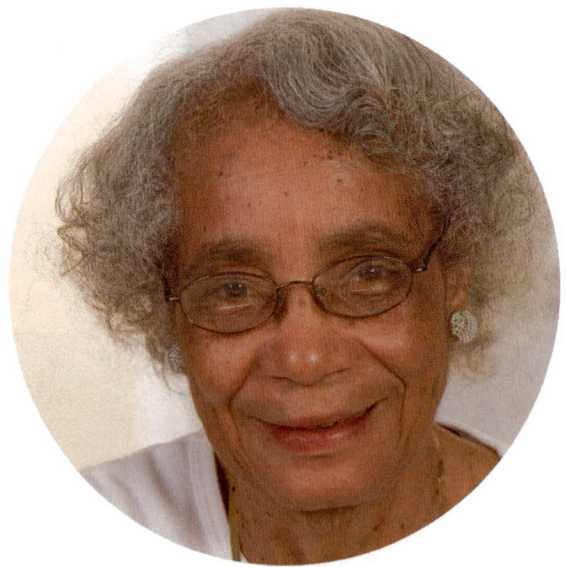

- **Talk about it.** Be open to hearing about feelings and memories. This is one of the most precious benefits of singing old familiar songs together. Invite conversation by asking questions, but don't put people on the spot. Keep in mind that for people with memory loss, being asked questions may be frustrating—and answering may not even be possible. If you sense frustration, let it go and move on.

- **Don't be afraid of sadness and tears.** There will be songs that make people feel sad. Music creates opportunities for people to express grief and for you to offer comfort. Don't be afraid of this. Allow people to express sorrow, and acknowledge them by saying something like, "You have such wonderful memories, don't you?" Then switch to a song with an upbeat tempo and positive message to help everyone change gears.

- **Change happens.** Our moods change, our energy levels change, and our brains change—especially in someone with dementia. This will show up in your music session. When it does, it's up to YOU to be flexible.

- **The right way? The wrong way? It's all ok!** The purpose of these suggested activities is to help you connect. Unless you push people to do something they don't want to do, there is no way to goof this up.

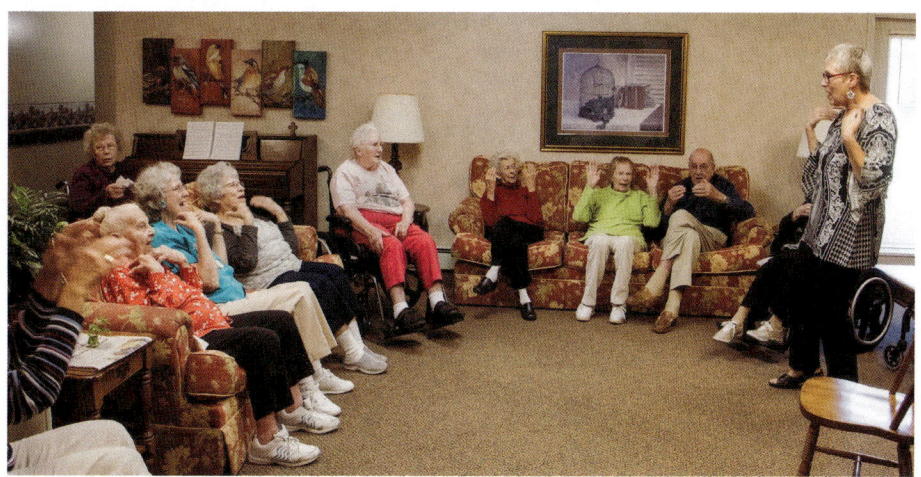

Music Moment with Mary Sue

Patty was the "life of the party" today. I thought she was going to bounce out of her chair. She has such great enthusiasm, and she has such a great sense of time. She was weaving and bobbing in the chair and tapping her toes and smiling and clapping along with syncopated rhythms, all at the same time! When we sang "Zippa Dee Doo Dah," she ended it with "Zippa dee doo dah, I've got a Blue Jay," while she patted her shoulder. We all laughed so hard. Sally, who had been telling me how depressed she has been, was laughing so hard the tears were running down her cheeks.

Patty is somewhat confused and is convinced that she had hired me to come sing with the ladies. She remarked, "I knew the ladies would enjoy this. It's easy to be down, but this lifts us up and this makes us happy. When you get to be our age, there aren't very many things that make us happy, but occasionally there'll be something that is a pleasant experience." Her friend Sally followed up by saying, "I haven't felt this good in a long time."

As I left, Patty told me, "I think the ladies really enjoyed it. I know how to get a hold of you. We'll have you back."

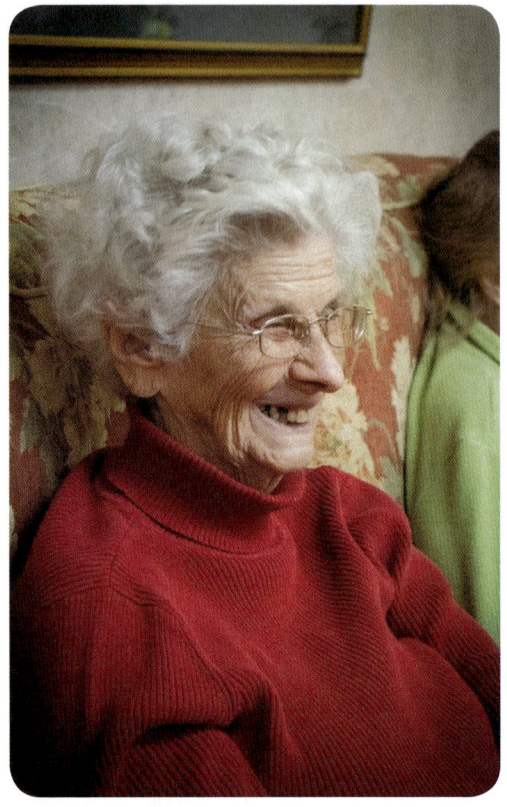

"For four hours on Wednesday nights, I offer my mom respite by sitting with my dad, who has Alzheimer's. I'm always seeking ways to connect with him. I'm happy to report that I found an amazing way to connect with my dad through Mary Sue's CD. I was amazed at my dad's ability to name the songs and sing along with the music. It brought such joy to our evening together."

Kelly Beischel, Daughter

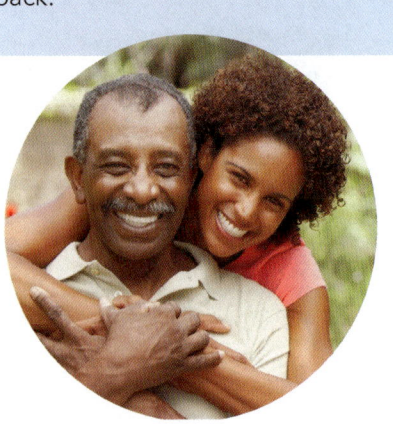

What if

They think I'm silly. Actually they probably won't. Our bodies naturally respond to music. Even people with late stage dementia will tap their toes and fingers to a steady beat.

They don't want to do it. That's OK! See if you can figure out why. Could it be the song selection? Are they introverts who don't enjoy group activities? If you are leading movement, they may prefer to simply sing along. They may prefer to just listen. Watch for small cues and slight movements. Sometimes all you will see is a tiny toe tapping.

I can't sing! No worries! Just sing anyway. This isn't a competition. Your enthusiasm will help others get started. The benefits of singing with someone do not depend on the quality of your voice. It would be a sad world if all mothers had to audition before they sang to their babies.

"My grandfather struggled with Alzheimer's in some of the last years of his life. During that time, it was amazing to witness the power of Mary Sue's music at work. These songs put that spark back in my grandfather's eyes. Even when simple tasks became incredibly difficult for him, Mary Sue was always able to get him singing and dancing. *Songs You Know By Heart* will get you doing the same."

Savannah Buist, Granddaughter

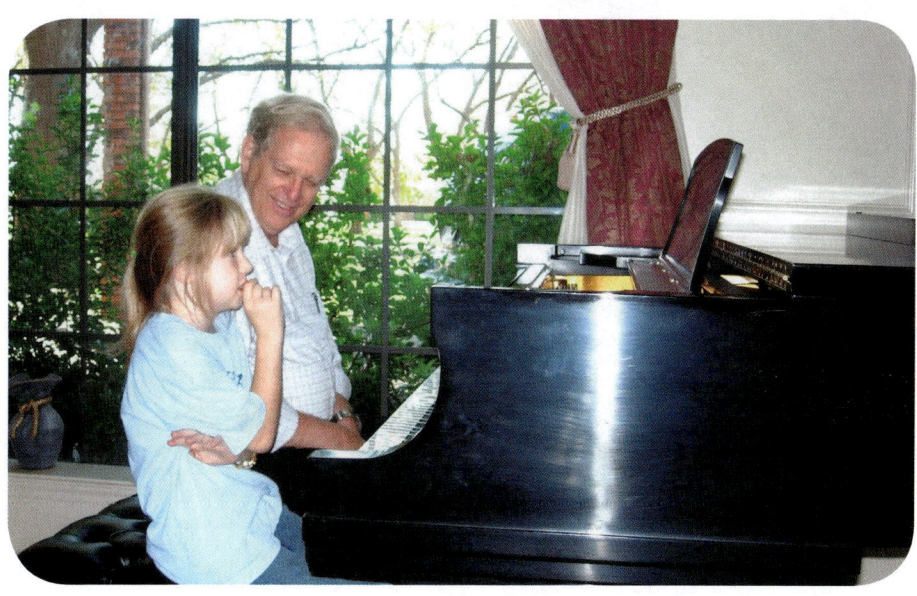

LET'S GET STARTED

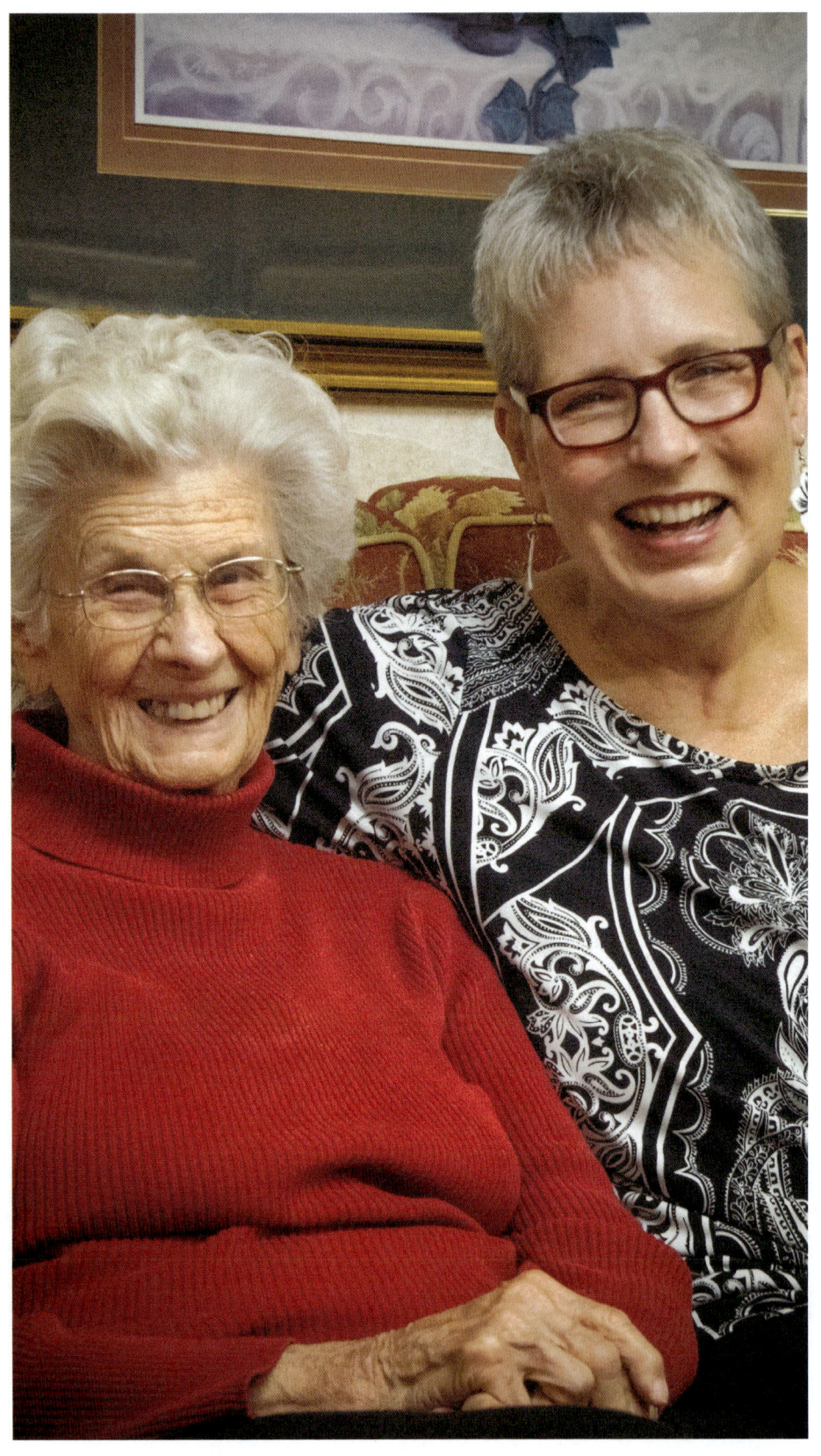

Chapter 3

Let's Sing!

Trust me when I tell you this: **everyone can sing**. Singing is as basic as walking and talking. People may say they can't sing, but when they hear a familiar song from their youth? Almost everyone will join in—especially if you are singing, too!

If possible, **listen to the songs ahead of time** so you can plan which ones to include and whether to use movement or discussion starters.

Decide if you will print copies of the lyrics. You may be surprised that some people with dementia can still read. For them, having the song lyrics helps a great deal. For others, it causes frustration and embarrassment. If you have the luxury of sitting side by side, you can point to lines of a song as you sing along.

> The fine print: Many songs fall under the category of Public Domain—making it legal to print and copy them as you please. These song lyrics are available on the Singing Heart to Heart website, www.SingingHeartToHeart.com. They are ready to print as individual song sheets in large, bold text. For songs that are **not** Public Domain, I provided websites that allow printing of the lyrics for your personal use only.

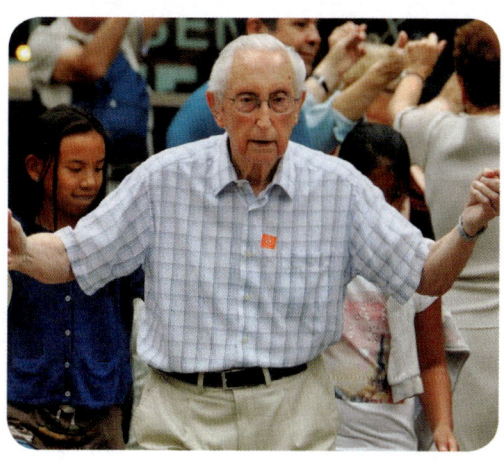

Music Moment with Mary Sue

Ron is asleep on the couch. When the singing starts he pounds one hand into the other in time to the beat. His eyes open now and then with what seems to be great effort. After some time Ron gets to his feet and comes to stand next to me. He starts to join in with a high-pitched hum. No words, just a hum in tune with the song. A hum and then a huge smile.

Ready, Set, Sing!

1. Begin with an upbeat song. Sometimes getting started is the hardest part. A lively song sets the stage. It's a good idea to vary the pace with one or two slower songs, but, overall, keep a singing session upbeat.

2. What's the name of this song? Everyone likes to know what's coming next. Begin with "How about we sing _____?" You can also sing the first words of a song and encourage them to finish the line. This is great fun and makes people with memory loss feel competent. It also gets them ready for what's next. For example: "My Bonnie Lies Over the _____." When they answer, be supportive with comments such as, "I knew you'd know this song!"

3. Sing along! Whenever possible, join in. Your participation is important. Singing together will help people feel like they belong.

4. Use movement on the first song. Adding movement right away gets things going and wakes everyone up.

5. Be positive! Encourage with comments such as, "We sound great today!" Add an enthusiastic thumbs-up gesture along with your great big smile.

Keep in Mind

- Our voices tend to get lower as we age. Keep the pitch lower.
- Don't sing too fast.
- Remember that repetition is ok. Sing songs more than once and on many occasions.
- Reluctant singers will often join in and continue singing with you if you begin with a patriotic song, such as "God Bless America."
- Take requests. What do THEY want to sing?
- Be a cheerleader and have fun!

Choosing Songs

How do you choose songs? Find out what people like.* If it's not possible to ask people directly or to interview their family, see if you can find out their age. Then count back through the decades so you can research what music was popular during their teens, twenties, and thirties. A simple online search for popular music by decade will get you started.

Additional characteristics of good sing-along choices:

- Songs with a strong, steady beat, such as "I've Been Working on the Railroad"
- Simple lyrics that repeat, such as "The Irish Lullaby"
- Songs with uplifting lyrics, such as "The Red, Red Robin"
- Funny songs, such as "The Old Gray Mare"
- Old folksongs that have been sung for generations, such as "Old McDonald Had a Farm"
- Patriotic songs, such as "God Bless America"
- Songs of faith and hymns, such as "In the Garden" and "Swing Low, Sweet Chariot"

* My e-book, *Finding Memories Through Music: A Family Interview*, contains a helpful interview guide and several suggested song lists. It can be purchased at www.SingingHeartToHeart.com. The website also has additional song lists and more activity suggestions.

Six Simple Songs to Sing

"Hail, Hail the Gang's All Here"

"I've Been Working On the Railroad"

"Let Me Call You Sweetheart"

"Take Me Out to the Ball Game"

"You Are My Sunshine"

"Goodnight Ladies"

Two Songs to Keep in Your Back Pocket

When you're stumped, rely on these two songs and the tips provided. One song will help you get things going again. The other will have a calming and soothing effect.

"I've Been Working on the Railroad"

Are people sitting around looking bored? Launch into this song and soon they will be singing with you and tapping their toes. This song has a strong, steady beat, and the lyrics are so well known that almost anyone can sing along. Use it when you want to create energy, motivate, or encourage movement. Don't hesitate to sing it more than once.

Encourage movement! Invite people to follow your lead as you pat your knees, tap your toes, etc. But don't get pushy—pat on your own knees, not theirs. Ensure their success by being mindful of what they're physically able to do. Accept their response or lack of response. Some may show only slight movements. Others may become leaders. If they are disinterested, they will let you know. Don't give up. Just try it another time.

This song is a march. Use its rhythm to motivate someone to walk with you from one place to another. But just hum the melody when using it this way. Otherwise, you are asking people to do two things at once, which may be hard for them.

Sing this song to "distract" and ease tension around an unpleasant task, such as showering.

Need to encourage a sleepy person to eat? Use this and other rousing songs a half hour before mealtime.

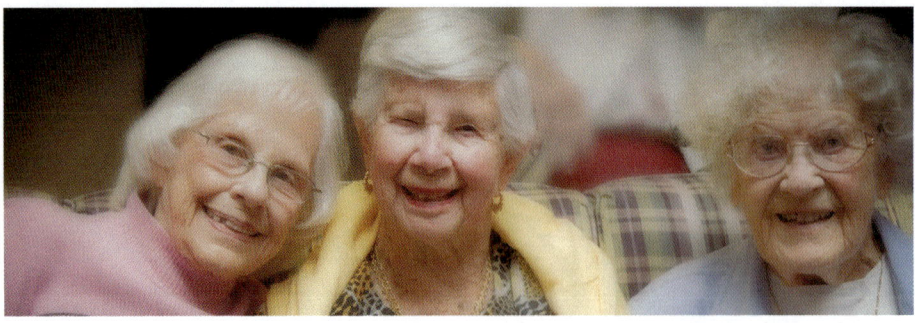

"Irish Lullaby" ("Too-ra-loo-ra-loo-ra")

What could be more soothing than a lullaby reminding you of your mother? "Irish Lullaby" is guaranteed to have a calming effect, especially if you sing it many times through. The words repeat, and almost everyone knows it. Don't worry about the verses; just sing the chorus. This song may well stir up an emotional memory. If it appears to make someone too sad, you may want to find a different lullaby.

Demonstrate and invite people (with gestures if necessary) to sway gently to the music, side to side with their shoulders or by waving their arms (as if directing a choir). With some people, you might see only a slight movement of the head. That's ok, too.

If possible, sing while rocking. Rocking affects the vestibular system and calms the central nervous system.

This song could be a perfect good night song or a cue for preparing for bed.

Nurturing is comforting. Provide a warmed towel, blanket, or beanbag for the person to cradle and rock as you sing with them.

Humming this song will also be calming. Humming creates vibrations in the mouth, and vibrations are soothing.

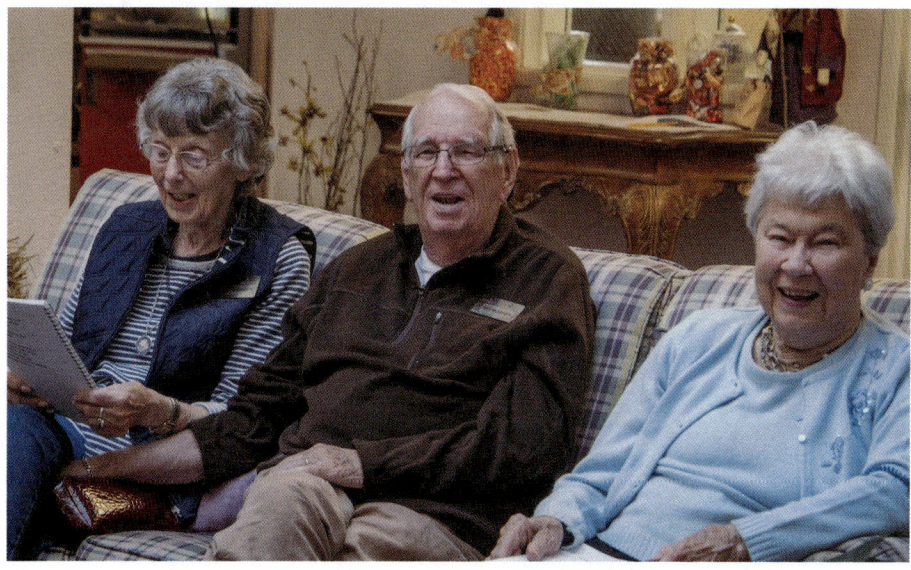

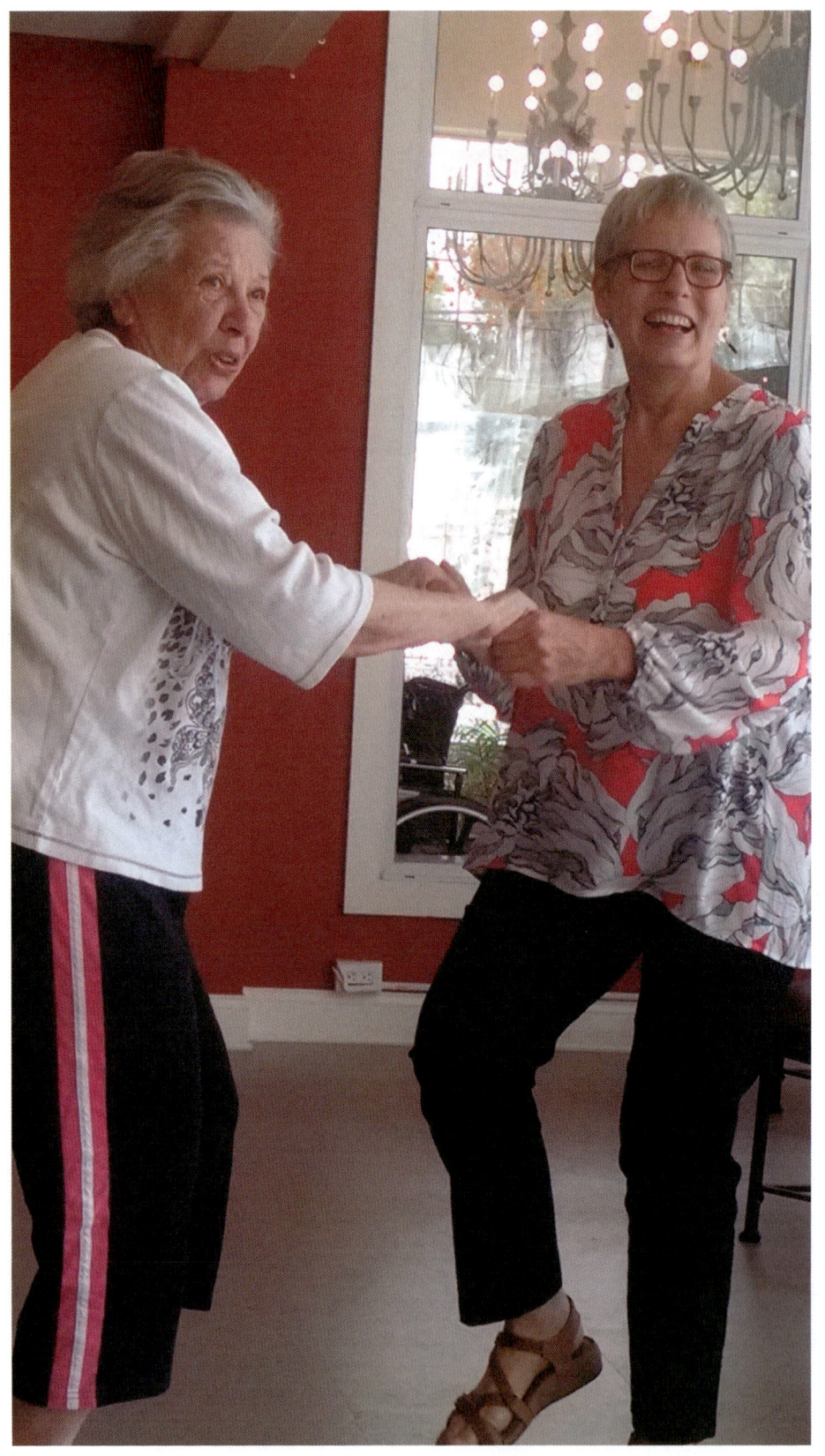

Chapter 4

Let's Move to Music!

Moving to music is possible for nearly everyone! And it's important because older adults can easily become sedentary. Most movements can be done sitting down, but don't hesitate to take to the dance floor if an individual is mobile. Some people with dementia may actually be able to dance better than they can walk.

Many people have limited range of motion. Adapt for this, and encourage them to do what is comfortable; nothing should cause pain. In a mixed group, some may be able to stomp their feet, while others are simply moving their toes.

The movements suggested in this chapter may seem simple, but they do provide much-needed exercise. They also add extra fun to a music session.

Will the music be fast or slow? Think about your goal. Are you hoping to energize people or provide movement to soothe them during an anxious moment.

Listen for the beat. Your choice of music will dictate the possible types of movement. An upbeat song calls for more active movements, while a lullaby suggests rocking, swaying, and peaceful breathing.

Mix it up. Keep things interesting by adding new movements, but stick to no more than two to four different movements for each piece of music.

Ready, Set, Move!

1. Animate and exaggerate. Use big gestures and make large movements with your body when you are demonstrating. Visual cues are the best way to give information. Make lots of eye contact and use their names frequently. Say *"Watch me and do what I do."*

2. Help them get started. People with dementia often have a hard time starting. Your movements will help them see what to do. If they seem engaged but don't follow your lead, offer your hands to them and gently move to the music. You will find that they often respond and carry on the movement once you get them going.

3. Go easy, from top to bottom. Start with an easy upper body movement, such as patting knees. Then add a lower body movement, such as toe tapping. Stay with one movement long enough for everyone to have some success—but not so long that arms or legs get too tired. Some instrumental music, especially Irish music and fiddle tunes, will have what are called A and B sections. You can use these as additional auditory cues for changing movements.

4. Anchor the beat and the movement by saying descriptive words in time to the music. For example: "March, march, march, march" or "Pat, pat, pat, pat."

5. Observe what they are able to do and adjust accordingly. Creating action sequences that are too complicated or too fast may be discouraging and make people feel incompetent.

6. Consider adding props to inspire movement and fun.

> ### Music Moment with Mary Sue
> Ellen wandered around, bending down to clean up tiny bits of dirt on the floor with her fingers. When the music started, Ellen's amazing sense of rhythm kicked in. She stepped side to side in time to the music, a huge smile plastered on her face. The music gave Ellen a way to express herself and to interact with the others. She could leave the bits of dirt on the floor and enjoy something she has been doing her whole life—dancing.

Props

- **Chiffon scarves** help people "dance" in their chairs or around the room as they wave the scarves. Playing with chiffon scarves to slow, fluid music is way more fun than you might think. They can be waved up and down, side to side, thrown in the air, or held at either end. Explore! And yes, both men and women enjoy this.

- **Egg shakers** are simple percussion instruments shaped like eggs. They are easy to hold and simple to use. Encourage people to shake them near their ears at first so they can hear the sound. Then lead other shaking movements—up high, down low, side to side, etc. After you're done, spray them with a disinfectant. You can buy them at music stores or online at sites such as Oriental Trading.

- **Straws or chopsticks** can be used like a conductor's baton. Simply tell people "Be the conductor!" A recorded version of "Stars and Stripes Forever" by the United States Marine Band is perfect for this but other songs will work too.

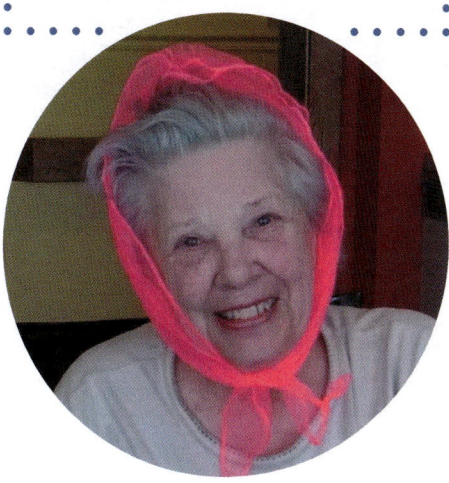

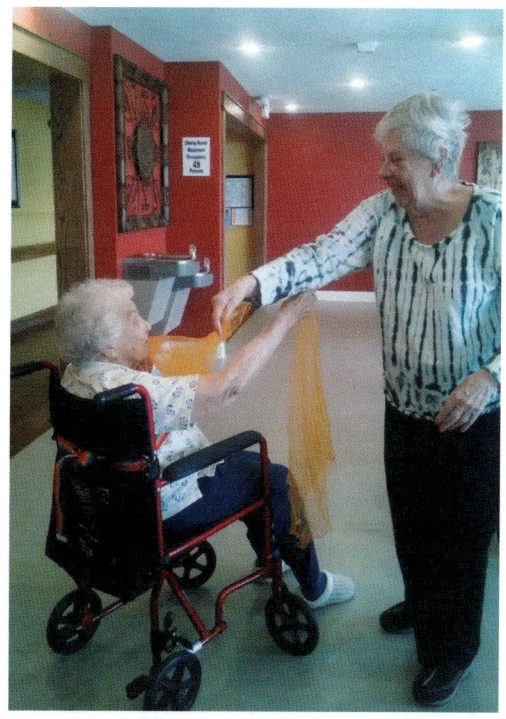

Music Moment with Mary Sue

As the Hawaiian music is playing, Joan arrives in her wheelchair. She's in a good mood and immediately starts to roll the chair around to the music. Betsy and I have already been dancing on our feet, and we join Joan in a sort of conga line as she circles around the tables. I hand out the chiffon scarves, do a two-second demonstration of waving them to the music, and off we go.

Joan is now up on her feet, dancing and swirling the scarves above her head, around in circles, and all around the room. Betsy gently drapes her scarf over Joan's head, and they both laugh. Everyone else is cheering us on. Joan says, "This is so much fun." I respond, "You're so much fun, Joan!" And we share a big hug.

Movement Ideas

Here are suggestions for some movements to try. What else can you think of? What spontaneous movements are people doing? Be a copycat!

Lower Body

- Tap your toes
- Tap your toes side to side with your heels anchored to the floor
- Tap your heels while your toes stay in place
- March in place, alternating feet
- Stomp with one foot and then the other
- Kick out one foot at a time so your heel rests on the floor
- Alternate legs as you kick out
- Move one foot to the side, then the other to the side, and finally back to center while you say, "Out, Out, In, In!"

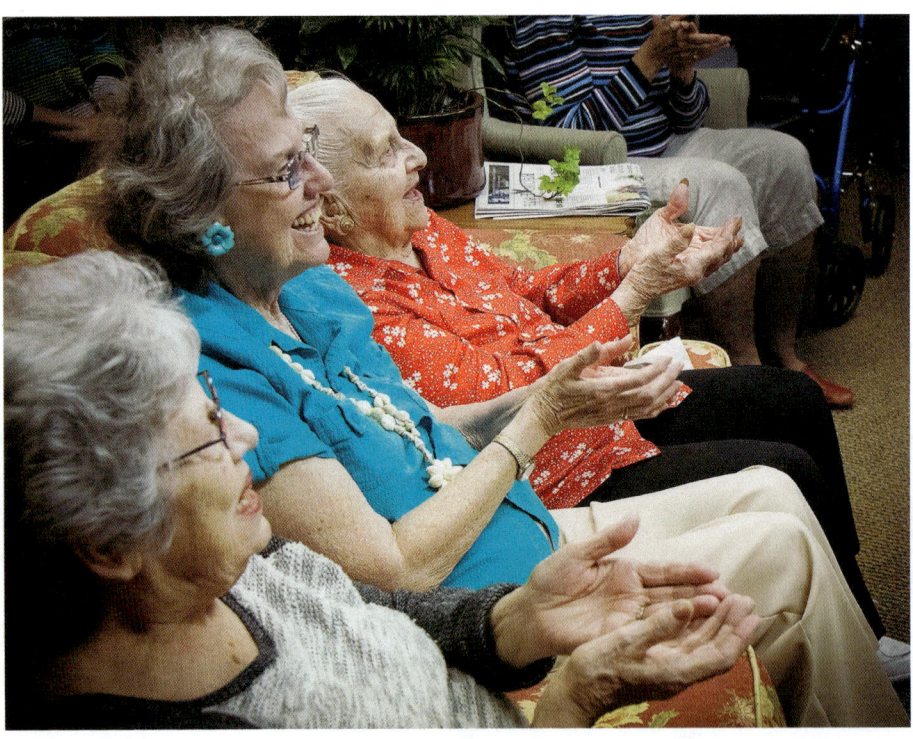

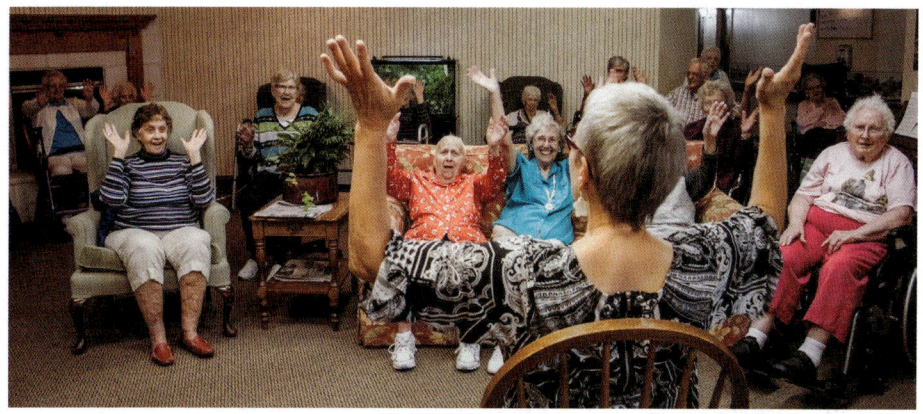

Upper Body

- Shrug shoulders up and down
- Clap hands in front
- Clap hands on one side of the body and then the other
- Clap hands high by your head and then lower toward your middle
- Clap hands making a circle in front of you
- Pat knees, pat shoulders, pat head
- Alternate between clapping hands and patting knees
- Do the "chicken dance," flapping your bent arms like wings
- Swing your arms from side to side (like waves)
- Extend your arms out straight and then bend them back so your hands touch your shoulders
- Extend fingers on both hands (like jazz hands) and move hands side to side
- Roll your hands and arms
- Extend your arms out to one side and then the other
- Raise your arms over your head while making a very excited face; then pull them in tight toward your body while making a grimace or funny face. You will look silly and so will they and this always gets a laugh!

A Simple 15-Minute Music and Movement Plan

The following are selections from Mary Sue Wilkinson's *Songs You Know By Heart* recording.

Track 1: "I Got Rhythm" (1:49) Use this song to lead off the session. It's lively and fun. Simply invite people to sing along!

Track 2: "Let Me Call You Sweetheart" (1:41) EVERYONE knows this song. Add a simple side-to-side wave with your arms or simply rock from side to side.

Track 3: "Don't Sit Under the Apple Tree" (1:33) This spirited World War II song is well known. It inspires knee patting and toe tapping. When you reach the lyrics "Don't go walking down lover's lane" in the second verse, add a walking movement while seated. And don't forget to wag your finger when "NO, NO, NO!" repeats.

Track 6: "My Bonnie Lies Over the Ocean" (2:43) During the verses, use your arms to make waves side to side (like ocean waves). At the chorus, extend your arms in front, then bend them back toward your shoulders as you sing "Bring back, bring back…"

Track 13: "Take Me Out to the Ball Game" (1:31) Batter up! Pretend to bat a ball and see if someone can guess what song you are going to sing. Then act out the song using your movements to keep time to the beat. Start the song "swinging" a bat, and shake a fist for "root, root, root for the home team." When you get to counting out the strikes, hold up one, then two, and then three fingers. Exaggerate the thumbs-up umpire's gesture for "You're Out!"

Track 17: "You Are My Sunshine" (2:36) This is a great song to end with. As you sing, add a simple hand or arm movement side to side. Try alternating between doing this above your head (or as high as they can reach)—as if your hands are the sun in the sky—and then at waist height.

One final hint: You can't do this wrong! Any movement is good. And, if someone in your group moves in a new way, don't hesitate to follow their lead.

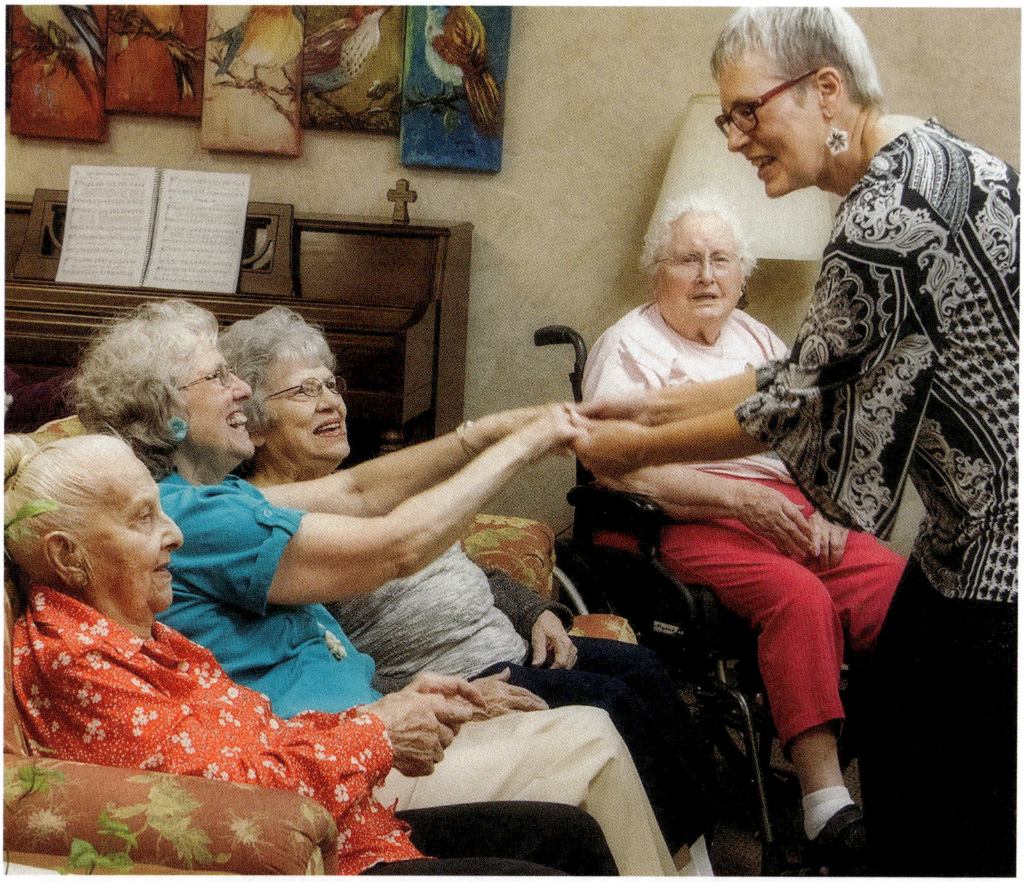

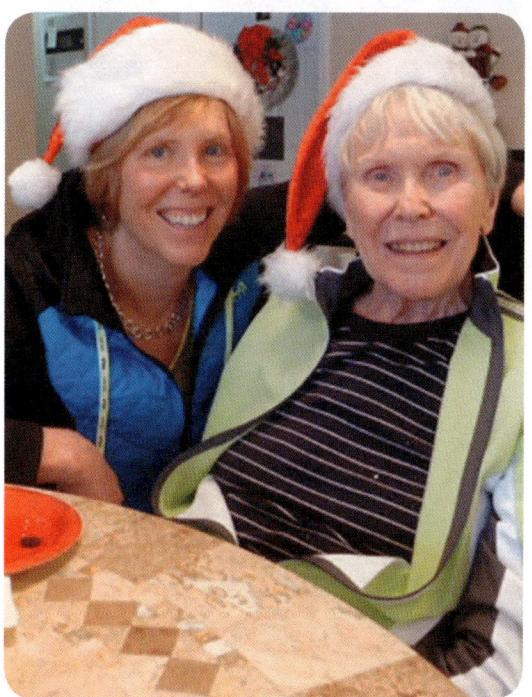

"When Mary Sue began singing with my mom and the residents where she lives, it enabled my mom to feel empowered, and it appeared to give her a lift in confidence that seemed to say "I can do this!" Since beginning with Young At Heart Music, I have seen a positive increase in my mom's ability to communicate with me. Because Alzheimer's disease and skill decline can be so cruel and difficult for family members to witness, it brings me great happiness to see such joy in my mom's face and mood."

Janet Ruggles, Daughter

LET'S MOVE!

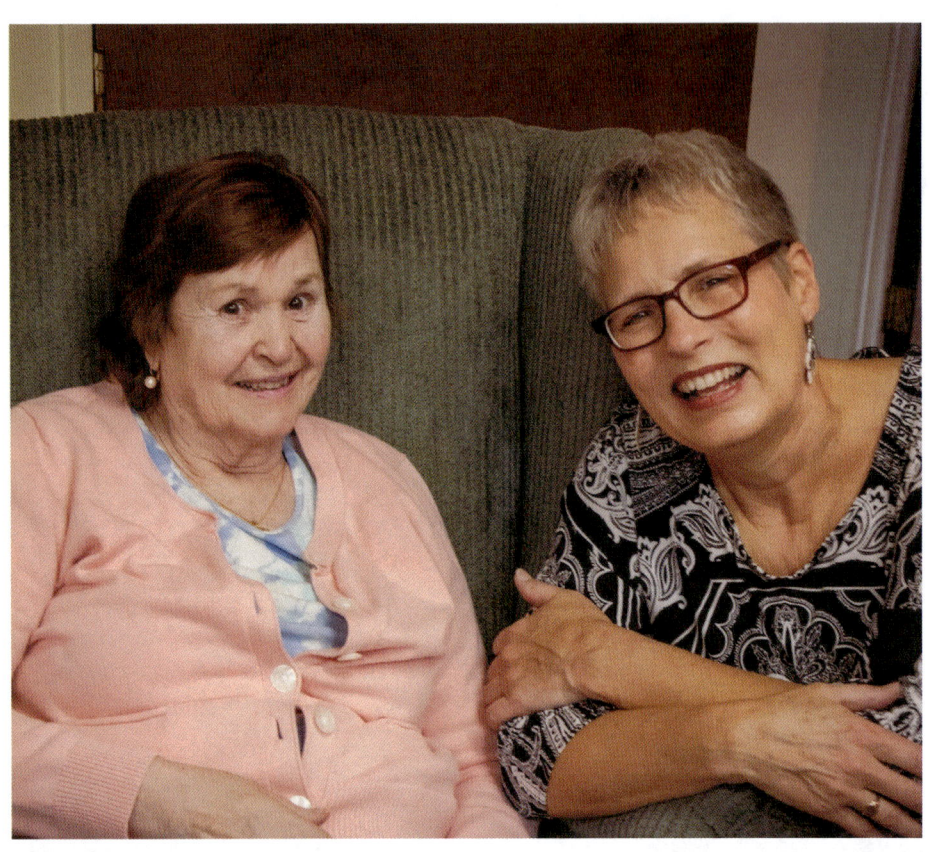
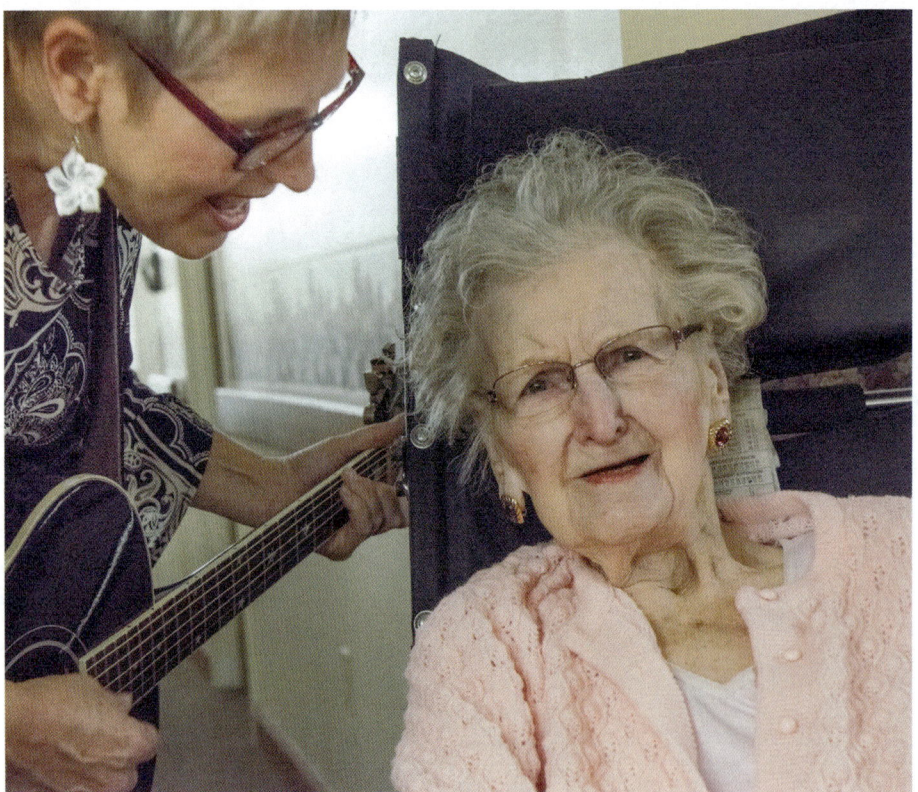

Chapter 5

Song by Song—
Using the *Songs You Know by Heart* Recording

Here are activity suggestions and discussion starters for each song, along with a little reminder about why music matters.

> To download all 18 songs from the CD head over to this private website page, **www.singinghearttoheart.com/songsforyou.** Enter the password "singing" to download your free copy of the CD. Additional copies of the physical CD are for sale on both Amazon.com and the Singing Heart to Heart website.

 Track 1: "I Got Rhythm" (George and Ira Gershwin) 1:49

Why? *Singing together creates a positive relationship.*

This familiar song is first on the CD for a reason. It inspires happiness. Play it at the beginning of each session, and it will soon be understood as a cue that it's music time. Snap your fingers; pat your knees; tap your toes; rock your body from side to side or even dance. Your enthusiasm will set the stage and encourage participation.

> **Talk about it/Music trivia**
>
> Do you like to dance? Did you see the movie, *An American In Paris*, that featured this song?

 Track 2: "Let Me Call You Sweetheart" (Friedman, Whitson) 1:41

Why? *Familiar songs provide a pathway to emotional memories.*

EVERYONE knows this song. Add a simple side-to-side wave with your arms or simply rock side to side. Because almost everyone will sing along to this song, consider focusing more on singing than on movement. Sometimes moving and singing at the same time are too hard.

> **Talk about it/Music trivia**
>
> This song was written in 1910! Who was your first sweatheart?

 Track 3: "Don't Sit Under the Apple Tree" (Stept, Brown, Tobias) 1:32

Why? *People remember songs from their youth.*

The words to this song repeat and are very similar verse to verse. Since the lyrics mention marching, try marching in your chair or around the room. Wag your finger whenever the words "No! No! No!" come around.

> **Talk about it/Music trivia**
>
> The Andrews Sisters performed this song during World War II. The message is: "Don't cheat on me!" Did any of your family members serve in World War II?

 Track 4: "Always" (Irving Berlin) 2:46

Why? *Music helps us link emotions to memories.*

This lovely waltz invites seated swaying from side to side or "waltzing" with your hands and arms in front of you.

> **Talk about it/Music trivia**
>
> This song was often featured at weddings. What was your wedding song? Do you know how to waltz?

 Track 5: "My Little Margie" (Conrad, Robinson, Davis) 1:53

Why? *People remember popular songs from their youth.*

This song has a bright tempo and lends itself to some chair dancing. See the suggested movements earlier in this chapter or make up your own. Use drumsticks, chopsticks, or even pencils as batons for "directing." Demonstrate a simple side-to-side motion with the "baton" and have everyone "direct" the song with you.

> **Talk about it/Music trivia**
>
> Of course, if there is someone named Margie, this is her song! Do you know anyone named Margie?

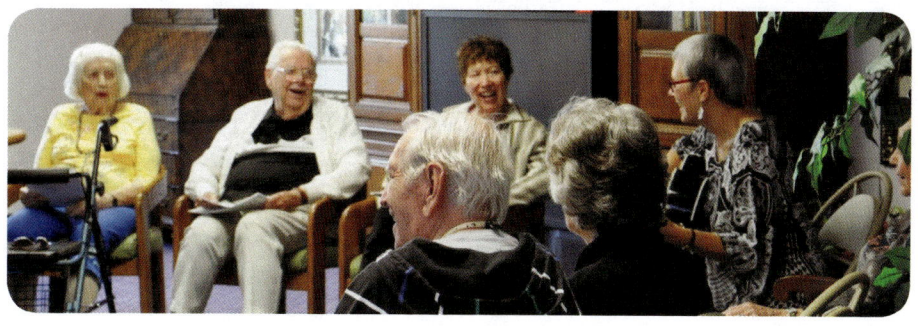

 Track 6: "My Bonnie Lies Over the Ocean" (Scottish Folk Song) 2:42

Why? *Songs can link us to childhood memories.*

This is an all-time favorite and should be on your short list of songs to keep in your back pocket. People never seem to tire of it. The song is so well loved and remembered that it reaches people at almost all stages of dementia. It's easy to add simple movements. Wave your hands in front of you as you sing the verses, as if making waves. At the chorus ("Bring back, bring back…"), extend your arms out and pull them toward you—as if you are actually bringing someone back to you. You can start by saying, "Watch me and do what I do."

> **Talk about it/Music trivia**
>
> Is anyone Scottish? This is a Scottish folk song.

 Track 7: "Peg O' My Heart" (Bryan, Fisher) 2:17

Why? *Music is not lost, even when other skills change.*

If people are mobile, this song has an easygoing tempo for dancing. It's also a good option for utilizing egg shakers or other simple percussion instruments. There are lots of words to the song and many may be forgotten. Most people come back to the lyrics "Peg of My Heart." It's ok if that is all you sing!

> **Talk about it/Music trivia**
>
> Is anyone Irish? Peg is the nickname for what names? (Margaret, Peggy)

 Track 8: "Bicycle Built for Two" (Dacre) 1:32

Why? *Singing familiar songs makes a person feel competent.*

Everyone knows the first verse to this song. They will probably not know the second verse about Harry. In the second verse, she tells him she's not crazy about him, and if he can't afford a carriage, there won't be any marriage!

> **Talk about it/Music trivia**
>
> Do you think she should have turned him down? Have you ever ridden a bicycle built for two?

 Track 9: "Four Leaf Clover" (Dixon, Woods) 1:42

Why? *Singing familiar songs makes people happy.*

This lively song has been known to get even shy singers to join in. Sing it with gusto! Add egg shakers or other hand-held rhythm instruments if you like. This is actually a slow polka, so if folks are steady on their feet and like to polka, it works well for dancing, too.

> **Talk about it/Music trivia**
>
> Have you ever found a four leaf clover?

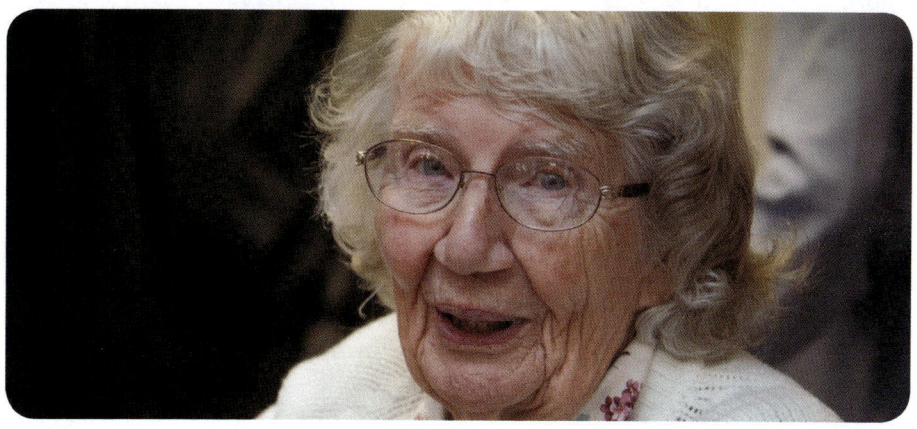

 Track 10: "Five Foot Two" (Lewis, Young, Henderson) 2:02

Why? *Rhythm remains as other abilities change.*

This is another all-time favorite, although most people will stumble a bit with the words unless they are using a songbook. Lead a chair dance. Kick one leg out with heel to ground and then the other. Alternate feet or stay on one side until everyone is with you; then switch. Don't go too fast. Use your arms to push out to each side, and open and close your hands twice on each side, as if you are trying to shake something off your fingers. This mimics what a flapper dancer might have done. Exaggerate the line "Bet your life it isn't her!"

> **Talk about it/Music trivia**
>
> Did you ever dance to this song?

 Track 11: "Shine on Harvest Moon" (Bayes, Norworth) 1:38

Why? *People can recall the words to familiar songs.*

Introduce this song by reviewing the lyrics. Say the first few words and have people finish the line. This is a great way to remind them of the words; it also makes people who are struggling with memory loss feel competent because they are finishing the line for you. Sway in time to the music. Many people really enjoy saying, "January, February, June, or July" with emphasis!

> **Talk about it/Music trivia**
>
> Let's say all the names of the months, beginning with January!

 Track 12: "(Put Another Nickel In) Music, Music, Music" (Weiss, Baum) 2:04

Why? *Music makes us want to move!*

Choose some lower body movements for a chair dance to this song. Egg shakers or other percussion instruments also work well for this energetic tune.

> **Talk about it/Music trivia**
>
> Who remembers what a nickelodeon is? Kids these days don't even know what a jukebox is, let alone a nickelodeon!

 Track 13: "Take Me Out to the Ball Game" (Norworth, Von Tilzer) 1:30

Why? *People can recall words to familiar songs, even when other memories are lost.*

Batter up! Pretend to bat a ball and see if they can guess what song you are going to sing. Then act out the song with movements in time with the beat. "Swing a bat" for the start of the song and shake a fist for "root, root, root for the home team." When you get to counting out the strikes, hold up one, then two, then three fingers and exaggerate the umpire's thumbs-up movement for "You're out!"

> **Talk about it/Music trivia**
>
> What's your favorite team? Are you a baseball fan? Insert the name of your favorite team in place of "home team." Did anyone watch the game last night? Who won?

 Track 14: "My Wild Irish Rose" (Olcott) 2:48

Why? *Songs provide a pathway to emotional memories.*

This is a pretty waltz that almost everyone knows and loves to sing. Enjoy! If you are with people who have sung a lot of harmony before, don't be surprised if they launch into beautiful harmonies on this song. Waltzes are always good songs for gently swaying back and forth.

> **Talk about it/Music trivia**
>
> Did you know this is just the chorus of a much longer song? It was featured in a movie by the same name in 1947.

 Track 15: "Sunny Side of the Street" (McHugh, Fields) 2:04

Why? *Singing happy songs makes you feel good.*

This is a great song for cheering people up. Get out the egg shakers if you have them or add some simple movements with arms and legs.

> **Talk about it/Music trivia**
>
> How rich was Rockefeller? Can you buy happiness?

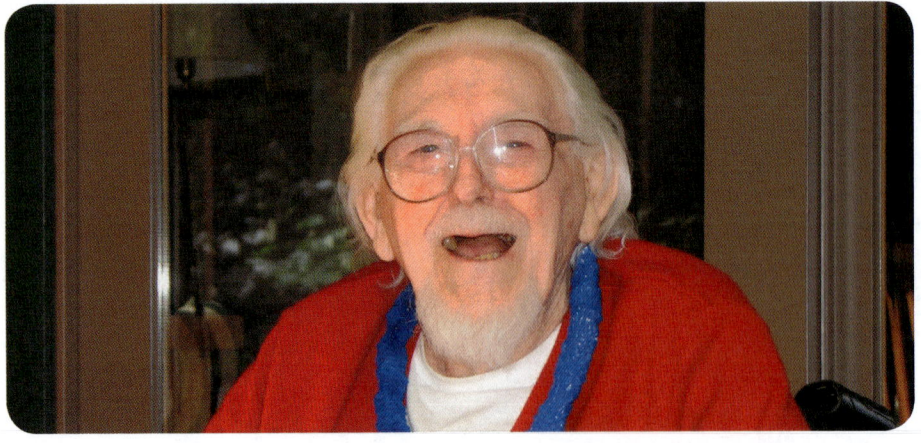

 Track 16: "Side by Side" (Woods) 2:13

Why? *Singing together creates community.*

The tempo of this song makes participation easy for people who have somewhat limited movement. Add some simple leg kicks or side-to-side action with your feet.

> **Talk about it/Music trivia**
>
> The question "Does anybody have a barrel of money buried in their back yard?" always brings a laugh. This song talks about how much more important togetherness is than money. Who's your best friend? Who was your best friend growing up?

 Track 17: "You Are My Sunshine" (Davis) 2:35

Why? *Singing familiar songs makes everyone feel comfortable and competent.*

A well-known song like this can be used throughout the day. Don't be surprised if people tell you they have sung this with their children. This is a good song to use at family gatherings because many young people also know it.

> **Talk about it/Music trivia**
>
> Did you know the Governor of Louisiana claims to have written this popular song? His name was Jimmie Davis. It's the state song and citizens called him their Singing Governor. Did you ever sing this with your family?

 Track 17: "When You're Smiling" (Shay, Fisher, Goodwin) 0:51

Why? *Music can lift your spirits!*

Lots of times older folks don't smile much. Just before I sing this one I say, "I'm looking for smiles." This is a great song to end a singing or music session.

> **Talk about it/Music trivia**
>
> Have you ever heard the expression "Fake it until you make it"? Do you think smiles are contagious?

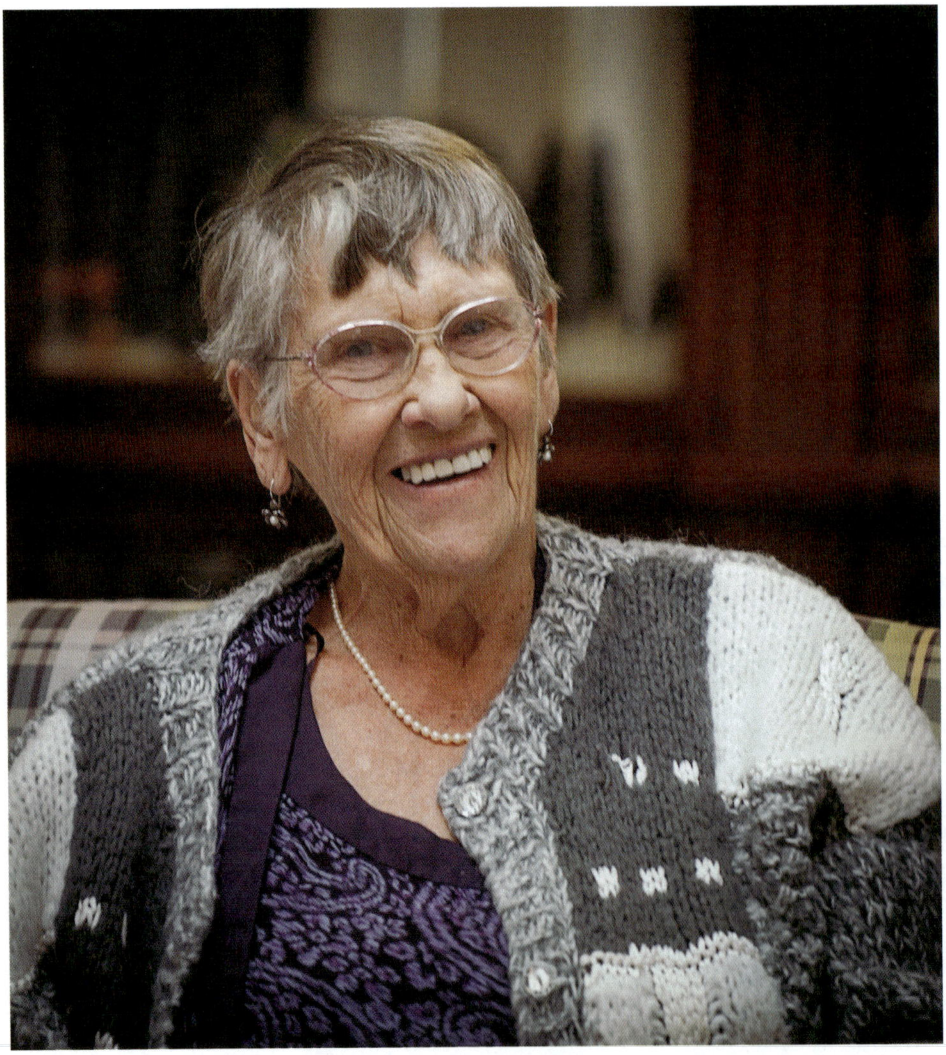

Your Notes

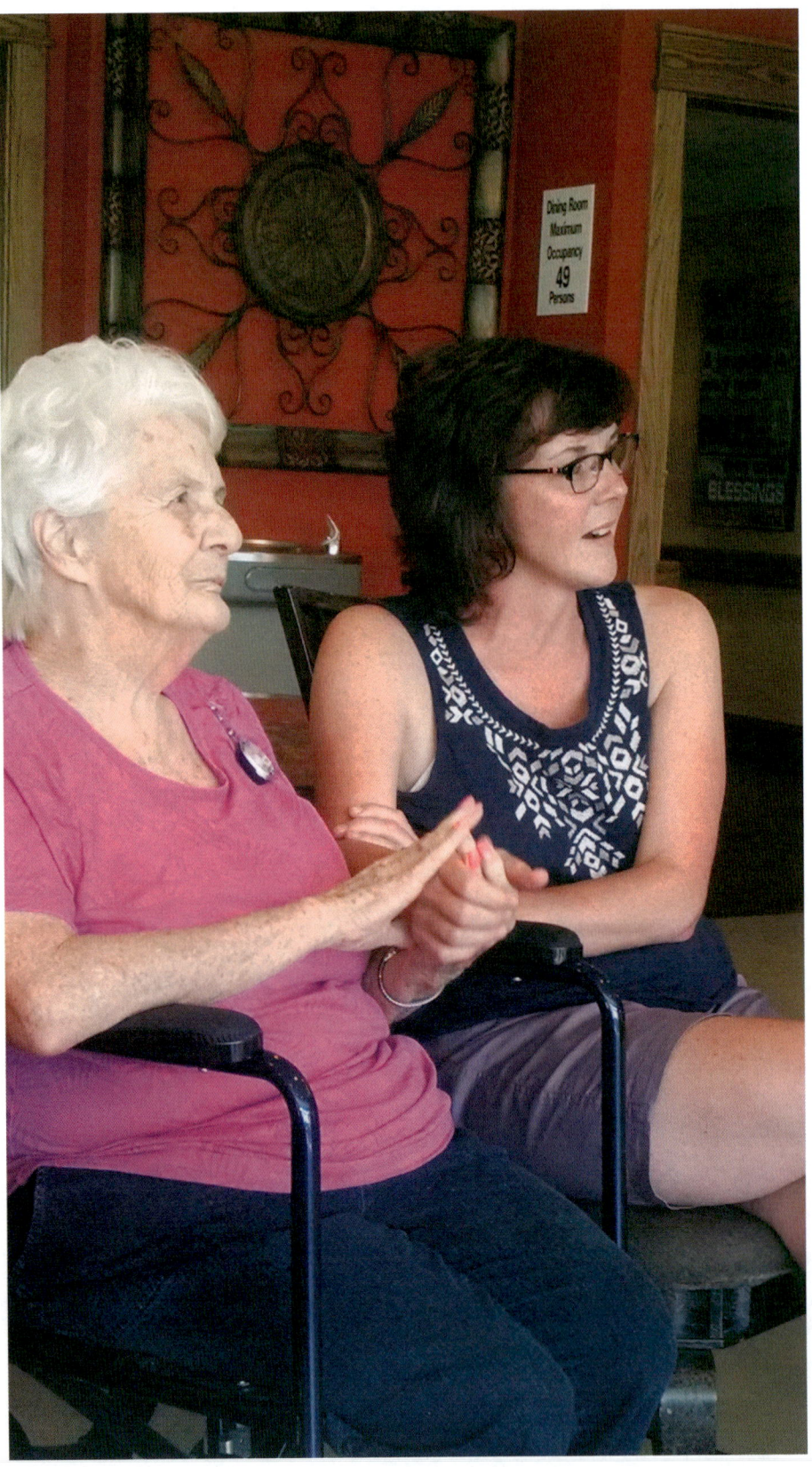

Chapter 6

Frequently Asked Questions

How long should a music session be?

It depends on the people in your care. Sessions could last from 10–45 minutes.

How often should I have music sessions?

Three or four short sessions throughout the day are recommended. Plan one longer 40–45 minute session daily if attention span allows.

I ask people if they want to sing and they say no. What do I do?

Invite, don't ask. Try saying, "Let's sing some songs," or "It's time to sing," or "Let's have some music!"

I play music in the background all day. Isn't that enough?

No! The goal is to use music to connect. A music session is about participation and engagement.

Sometimes I just need a break. Can't people sing with the CD on their own?

Yes, you can use the CD to provide an independent activity. But keep in mind that people with dementia often have a hard time beginning. Help them get started by singing with you, and then come back occasionally for a few lines, and show enthusiasm and encouragement.

How do I know what kind of music they will like?

Ask questions! Explore music from youth and childhood. The *Songs You Know By Heart* CD can help.

What's a good song to begin a music session?

If you are singing with an individual, try a song they love. It can become your "Here I am!" song to cue them that music time is starting. Many people love "You Are My Sunshine." If you are singing with a group, a good song is "Hail, Hail, the Gang's All Here."

What's a good song to end the session?

"Goodnight Ladies" or "When You're Smiling."

I don't have time to play a lot of songs. Are there a few that I can just sing when I feel like I need one?

"My Bonnie Lies Over the Ocean," "Take Me Out to the Ball Game," "I've Been Working on the Railroad," and "You Are My Sunshine" are good choices.

What if they don't want to sing or participate?

Don't give up too easily, but don't be pushy. It may be hard to see someone's response to the music, but unless they clearly let you know they don't like it, you can continue to play a few songs.

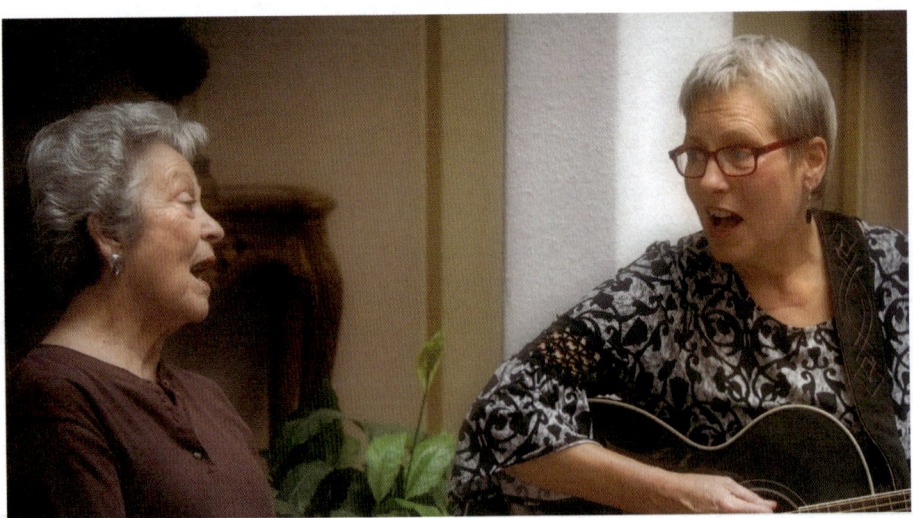

How many times through should I sing the same song?

At least twice, and more if they seem to be really enjoying it. Sometimes it takes one time through the song before people will join in.

Where should I sit?

If the individual is right-handed, sit toward the right side but make sure you can still be seen. Left-handed? Do the opposite. If you're singing with a group, you may want to be on your feet, moving around to provide encouragement and eye contact.

They don't seem like they are even listening. What do I do?

Respect personal space, but try to make eye contact and smile. Play and/or sing "My Bonnie Lies Over the Ocean." Kneel down so you can look up into someone's eyes. Offer your hands so you can share a gentle side-to-side movement in time to the music. Holding hands, swaying, eye contact, and this particular song seem to be a magical combination.

Where can I find the song lyrics?

The lyrics for my CD, as well as many others, are available at www.SingingHeartToHeart.com. For more songs, conduct a simple online search by typing in "lyrics for (fill in the blank)." There are numerous lyrics websites that will allow you to view and copy the words to thousands of songs.

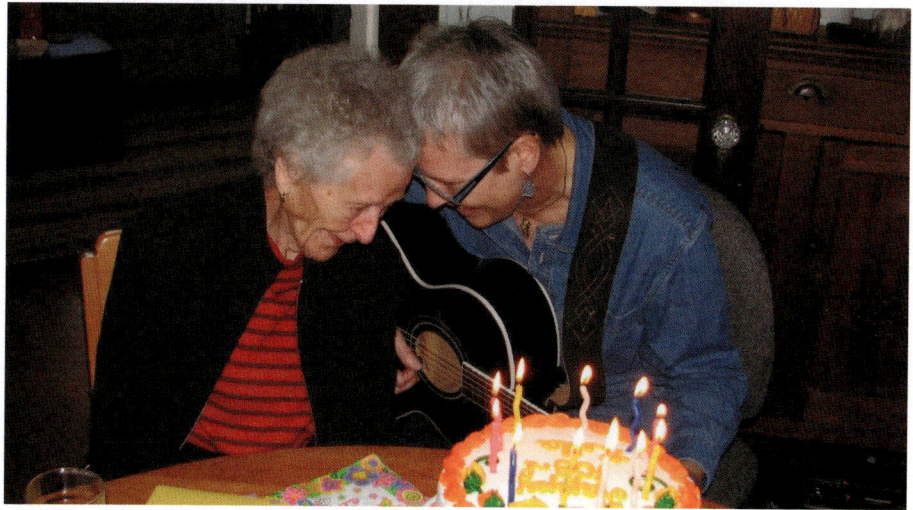

What's a good song for helping someone relax?

My favorite is "Irish Lullaby," which has a very repetitive chorus of "Too-ra-loo-ra-loo-ra." It's worth learning if you don't know it. You can find it at www.SingingHeartToHeart.com.

What's a good song to help someone go from one room to the next?

"Sentimental Journey" and "I've Been Working on the Railroad" are both good choices. Remember to hum the song. If you sing the words, the person you want to walk with you will probably stop to sing, rather than keep walking.

Are there any good songs to sing when young grandchildren visit?

Go ahead and sing the songs little ones enjoy. Older people will remember them too—and singing together helps everyone connect and enjoy the visit. "Twinkle Little Star," "ABC," "Baa Baa Black Sheep," and "If You're Happy and You Know It" are good choices.

Why do I have to sing along?

Singing together is the way you connect. Connecting is the goal!

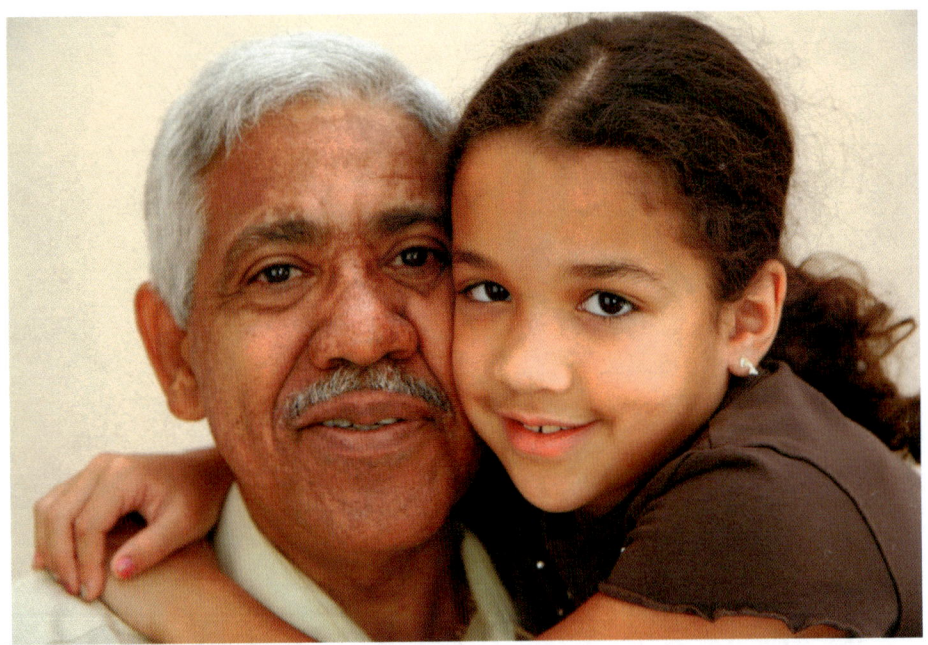

Won't they get bored singing the same songs all the time?

No! People with memory loss appreciate structure and routine. Their world is full of things they can't anticipate or understand. Mixing it up is fine, but always begin and end with the same songs—and don't hesitate to sing them over and over.

What's a good song to sing when people seem bored?

Pick something rousing. A happy song can really lift the mood. If you are singing on your own without the CD, try an old folk song, such as "Old MacDonald," "I've Been Working on the Railroad," or "Take Me Out to the Ball Game." If you are using the *Songs You Know by Heart* CD, try launching into Track 12 with "Music! Music! Music!" followed by tracks 13, 14 and 15.

I don't have a CD player. Now what?

Singing without the CD is "legal" and encouraged! Check out Chapter 3 for song suggestions and support.

How can we dance safely? I'm worried about falls.

Follow the individual's lead; he or she will show you what they can do. This is not the time to get fancy and show off your own dance moves. Simple side-to-side steps while holding hands is a good place to start. Backing up can be difficult, so keep moving forward. Do you have safety railings in the hallway they can hold on to? Be aware that those in your care may tire more easily than you do.

Why does the same song make one person happy and another person sad?

Songs are connected to deep emotional memories. We all have different experiences and memories.

I try to sing all the songs during music time, but I'm interrupted by a lot of talking. What do I do?

Shift to talking! One of the joys of using music is that it can awaken memories and give people an opportunity to share who they are and what they have done in life.

What's a good song for bath time?

It depends on the person. For some, adding relaxing instrumental music ("Blue Danube" and wooden flutes, for example) will help create a spa-like experience, as will soft lights and aromas of lavender or rose. For other people, you may need to use music to provide information about what is happening. For example, "I'm Gonna Wash That Man Right Out of My Hair" or "Splish Splash I'm Takin' a Bath." If you are a family member who is intimate with the person bathing, choose a well-loved and lively song. This helps the person who is being bathed focus more attention on your relationship than the mechanics of the bath.

I don't know all the words to these old songs, and they can't remember all of them either. What do I do?

Song lyrics for my CD are available at www.SingingHeartToHeart.com. But don't hesitate to randomly sing "la, la, la!" Some people will enjoy humming or just singing syllables.

The folks I work with can't do all that movement stuff. They're in wheelchairs and have arthritis. Now what?

All the movements can be adapted. There is no right or wrong way to move except to make sure no one is in pain. Just have fun!

I can't get people to do the movements the same way I do. How do I get them to follow me?

It doesn't matter if they follow you. Your goal is to introduce movement to the music. If they move in their own way, just follow their lead. Or you can say, "Let's try this!" Anchoring a movement with a word helps. For example, try saying, "March, march, march" or "Pat, pat, pat" to the beat of the music.

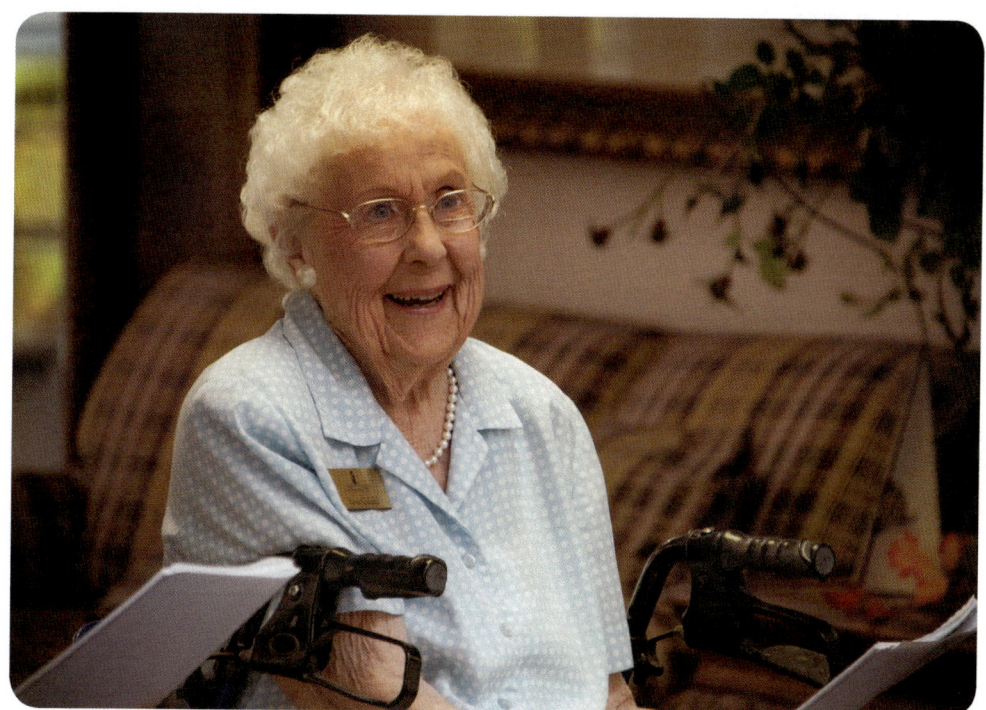

"I can't believe I remember all the words to these songs from my youth. How can that be? I haven't heard them in so many years!"

Lois, Assisted Living Resident

Music Moment with Mary Sue

Today I thought I would burst into tears of happiness. My eyes glistened and so did Margaret's. She usually prefers to use printed song lyrics, which she is still quite capable of reading. Today we were "going off program" and not using the lyrics.

I launched into "Shortening Bread" and Margaret joined me enthusiastically. The lyrics are: "Two little children lying in bed, one was sick, the other half dead, call for the doctor, doctor said—feed those children some shortening bread!" We got to laughing, and next thing I knew, Margaret was fairly coming out of her seat, clapping and laughing and singing, "Mama's little baby loves shortening, shortening!" We laughed even more.

I have felt happiness while singing before, but sitting side by side with Margaret today … well, it was as if an electrical current ran between us—almost in the same way you can feel communicating with your lover or your child. Pure joy!

FAQ

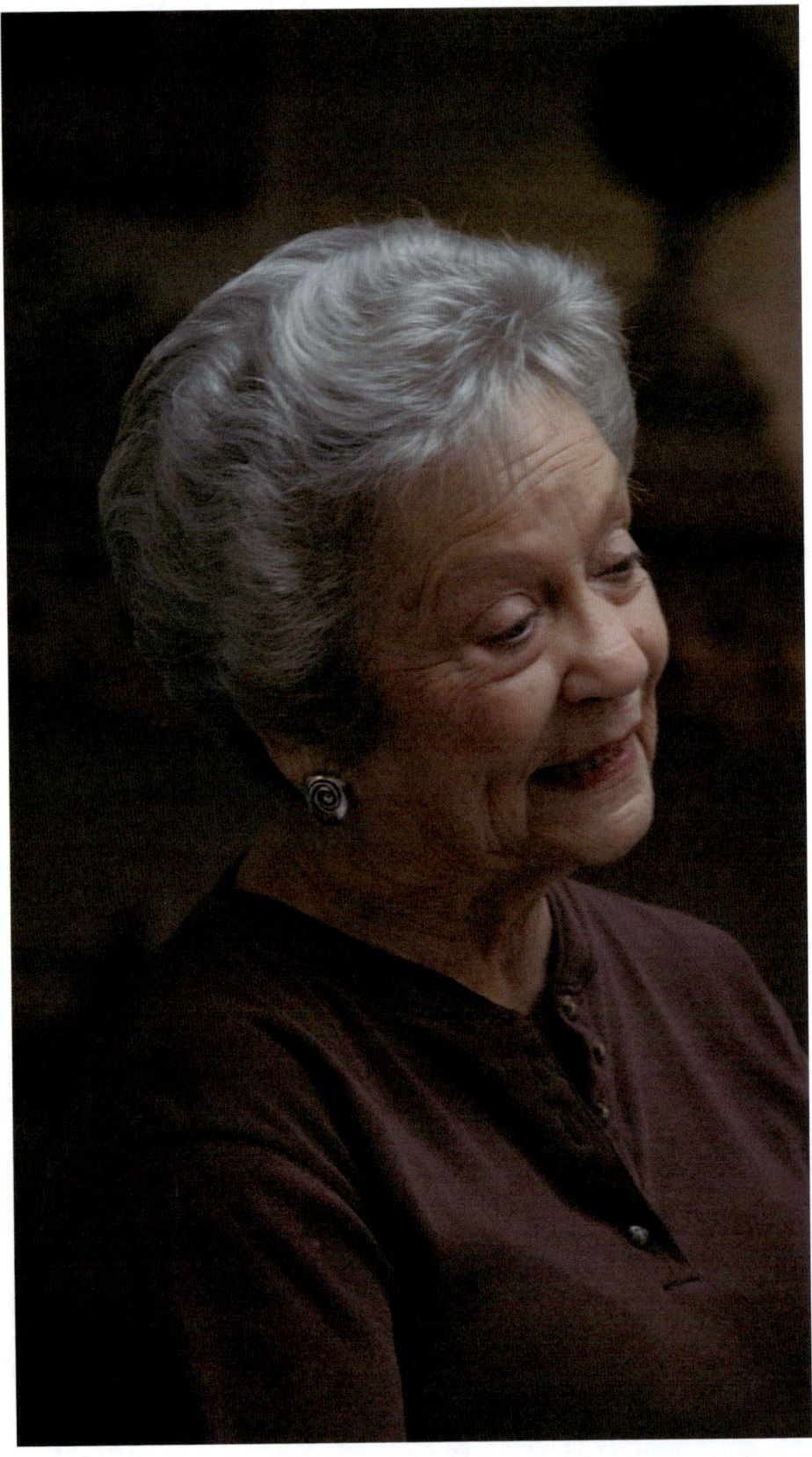

Chapter 7

Introducing Teepa Snow's GEMS™ Model

Note from the Author:

I first learned about Teepa Snow from an activity director at an assisted living home where I sometimes sing. The videos and resources I discovered on Teepa's website quickly revealed that the simple skills and strategies she teaches could help me do a better job engaging with people who are living with dementia and Alzheimer's.

Teepa is known as Today's Voice for Dementia. She is a leading advocate and educator worldwide for people living with dementia and Alzheimer's, as well as their care partners.

I reached out to Teepa, sharing my CD and telling her about the work I do. In March 2015, she invited me to audit her Consultant Certification Training. After hours of online training videos, studying, and digging deeper into the Positive Approach to Care and the GEMS model, I traveled to Nashville to train with Teepa in person.

This section introduces Teepa's groundbreaking GEMS dementia classification model. This model will help you understand the behavior of people living with dementia and Alzheimer's. Behavior is communication, especially after language is lost. GEMS is an important tool to have in your toolbox. I have learned a lot from it, and now you can too. I urge you to refer back to it frequently.

—Mary Sue Wilkinson

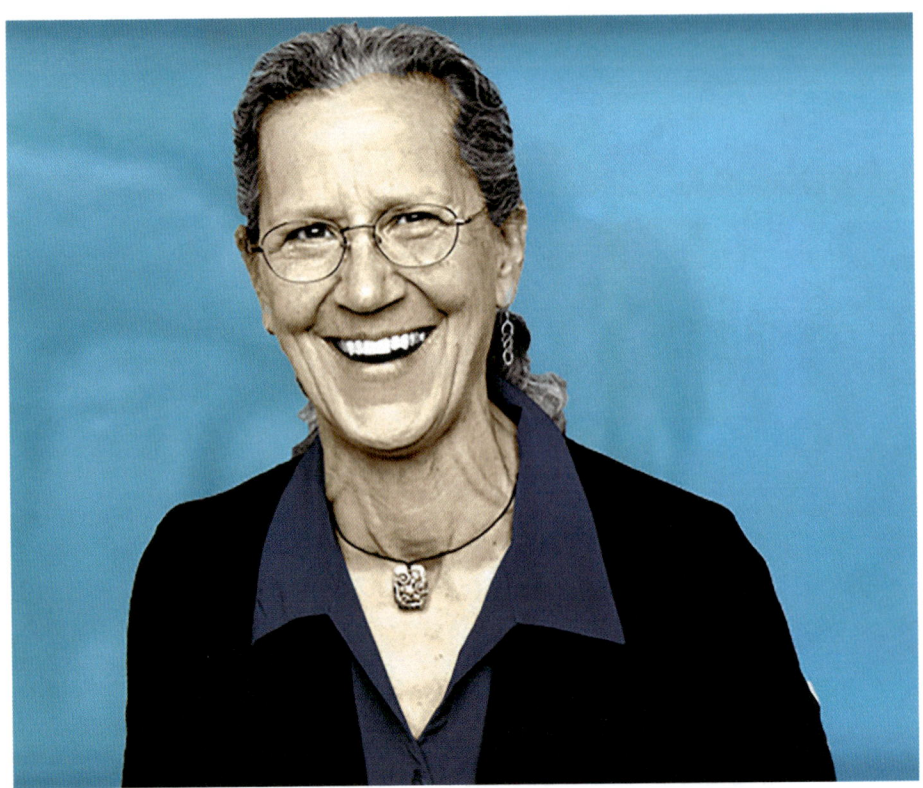

GEMS™

The GEMS dementia classification model revealed in this chapter recognizes the dynamic nature and abilities of the human brain. Unlike other cognitive models, it acknowledges that everyone's abilities can change in a moment. Modifying environments, situations, interactions, and expectations will either create supportive and positive opportunities or result in distress and a sense of failure.

Just as gemstones need different settings and care to show their best characteristics, so do people. Rather than focusing on a person's loss when there is brain change, seeing individuals as precious, unique, and capable encourages a care partnership. That is the core of this model. Providing supportive settings for everyone, including care providers, allows people to use what they have to be their best. The GEMS advocate that everyone living with brain change will shine when given the opportunity.

—Teepa Snow and Positive Approach™ to Care Team

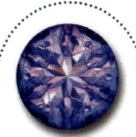

Sapphire - True Blue - Optimal Cognition, Healthy Brain

True to self; personal preferences remain basically the same

Can be flexible in thinking and appreciate multiple perspectives

Stress/pain/fatigue may trigger Diamond state;
returns to Sapphire with relief

Able to suppress and filter personal reactions;
chooses effective responses

Selects from options and can make informed decisions

Processes well and is able to successfully transition

Aging doesn't change ability; processing slows,
more effort/time/practice needed

My brain is healthy and true blue. If I am aging normally or I am distressed, it may be hard for me to find words. I can describe what I am thinking so you understand. I may talk to myself to give myself cues and prompts. I can learn new things and change habits, but it takes time and effort. Whenever possible, honoring my choices and preferences is important. I need more time to make decisions. Give me the details and let me think about it before you need an answer. I am able to remember plans and information, but supports are helpful. I may like specific prompts such as notes, calendars, and reminder calls. Changes in vision, hearing, balance, coordination, depression, anxiety, pain, or medication may impact my behavior—but my cognitive abilities remain the same.

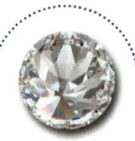

Diamond - Clear and Sharp - Routines and Rituals Rule

Displays many facets; behavior and perspective can shift dramatically

Prefers the familiar and may resist change; challenged by transitions

More rigid and self-focused; when stressed, sees wants as needs

Personal likes/dislikes in relationships/space/belongings become more intense

Reacts to changes in environment; benefits from familiar; functional/forgiving

Needs repetition and time to absorb new/different information or routines

Trusted authority figures can help; reacts better when respect is mutual

My overall cognition is clear and sharp. When happy and supported, I am capable and shine in my abilities. When distressed, I can be cutting and rigid and may see help as a threat. I have trouble seeing other points of view and may become less aware of boundaries, or more possessive about my relationships, personal space, and belongings. I have many facets so people see me differently depending on the situation. This can cause conflict among my family, friends, or care team, as it's hard to tell if I am choosing my behavior or truly have limits in my ability. I can engage socially and have good cover skills. People will vary in their awareness of what is happening to me. I want to keep habits and environments as they have always been, even if they are problematic for others or me. I am often focused on the past, personal values, or finances. I need help to make changes in my life; it's hard for me. I can be in a Diamond state for reasons other than dementia.

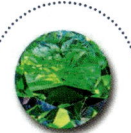

Emerald - Green and On the Go with a Purpose - Naturally Flawed

Sees self as able and independent with limited awareness of changes in ability

Lives in moments of clarity mixed with periods of loss in logic/reason/perspective

Understanding and use of language changes; vague words and many repeats

Cues and support help with getting to or from places or in doing daily routines

Awareness of time, place, and situation will not always match current reality

Strong emotional reactions are triggered by fears, desires, or unmet needs

Needs to know what comes next; seeks guidance and assistance to fill the day

I am flawed; it is part of being a natural emerald. I tend to be focused on what I want or need in this moment and may not be aware of my own safety or changing abilities. I can chat socially, but I typically miss one out of every four words and cannot accurately follow the meaning of longer conversations. I won't remember the details of our time together, but I will remember how your body language and tone of voice made me feel. I may hide or misplace things and then believe someone has taken them. My brain makes up information to fill in the blanks, which makes you think I am lying. If you try to correct me or argue, I may become resentful or suspicious of you. I am not always rational, but I don't want to be made to feel incompetent. My brain plays tricks on me, taking me to different times and places in my life. When I am struggling, I may tell you, "I want to go home." To provide the help and assistance I need, you must go with my flow—using a positive, partnered approach—and modify my environment.

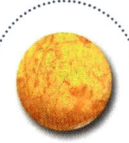

Amber - Caught in a Moment of Time - Caution Required

Focused on sensation; seeks to satisfy desires and tries to avoid what is disliked

Environment can drive actions and reactions without awareness of safety

Visual abilities are limited; focus is on pieces or parts, not the whole picture

What happens to or around an Amber may cause strong and surprising reactions

Enters others' space and crosses boundaries in attempt to meet own needs

Has periods of intense activity; may be very curious or repetitive with objects or actions

Care is refused or seen as threatening due to differences in perspective and ability

Like a particle trapped in an amber, I am caught in a moment of time. It may surprise you to see how I take in the world around me. I may not know you or see you as a whole person. I react to you based on how you look, sound, move, smell, and respond to me. I like to do simple tasks over and over; I may need to repeatedly move and touch, smell, taste, take or tear items apart. While it may exhaust or frustrate you, it soothes me. You have to safeguard my environment because I don't recognize danger. I'm intolerant to discomfort because my mouth, hands, feet, and genitalia are highly sensitive due to changes in my nervous system. Therefore, activities like eating, taking medication, mouth care, bathing, dressing, and toileting may distress me. Please notice my reaction and stop if I am resisting. I can't help myself, and one or both of us may get hurt emotionally and/or physically. If this happens, wait a few minutes, then connect with me and try a different approach—possibly substituting one area of focus for another.

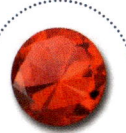

Ruby - Deep and Strong in Color - Others Stop Seeing What is Possible

Makes use of rhythm; can usually sing, hum, pray, sway, rock, clap, and dance

When moving can't stop, when stopped can't get moving; needs guidance and help

Big, strong movements are possible, while skilled abilities are being lost

Danger exists due to limited abilities combined with automatic actions or reactions

Tends to miss subtle hints, but gets magnified facial expressions and voice rhythms

Can mimic actions or motions, but will struggle to understand instructions/gestures

Able to pick up and hold objects, and yet not know what to do with them

As the deep red of a ruby masks its detail, my obvious losses make my remaining abilities harder to notice. Although my fine motor skills have become very limited, remember that I am able to move and do simple things with my hands. You need to anticipate, identify, and respond to all of my needs, even though I may not be aware of them. Plan to create a supportive environment, help with the details of care, and structure my day. Just as a crossing guard directs traffic, you must guide my movements and transitions. I can rarely stop or start on my own, and switching gears is a challenge. Move with me first, then use your body to show me what you want me to do next—one step at a time. Hand-Under-Hand™ assistance helps me to feel safe and secure and know what to do. Losses in visual skills, chewing abilities, balance, and coordination make danger a part of my life. You can reduce the risks to me but not eliminate them. I can still have moments of joy when you are able to provide what gives me pleasure.

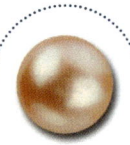

Pearl - Hidden Within a Shell - Beautiful Moments to Behold

Will frequently recognize familiar touches, voices, faces, aromas, and tastes

Personhood survives, although all other capabilities are minimal

Understanding input takes time; go slow and simplify for success

In care, first get connected by offering comfort; then use careful and caring touch

Changes in the body are profound; weight loss, immobility, systems are failing

As protective reflexes are lost, breathing, swallowing, and moving will be difficult

Care partners benefit from learning the art of letting go rather than simply giving up

While hidden like a pearl in an oyster shell, I still have moments when I become alert and responsive. I am near the end of my life. Moments of connection create a sense of wholeness and value between us. Use our time together not just to provide care but also to comfort and connect with me. To help me complete life well, it's important to honor my personhood when making medical or care decisions; please don't talk about me as though I am not still here. I respond best to familiar voices and gentle rhythmic movements. I am ruled by reflexes and startle easily. My brain is losing its ability to control and heal my body. Be prepared to see me having difficulty breathing or swallowing. My body may no longer desire food and drink as I prepare to leave this life. I may not be able to stop living without permission from you. Your greatest gift at this time in my life is to let me know that it is okay to go.

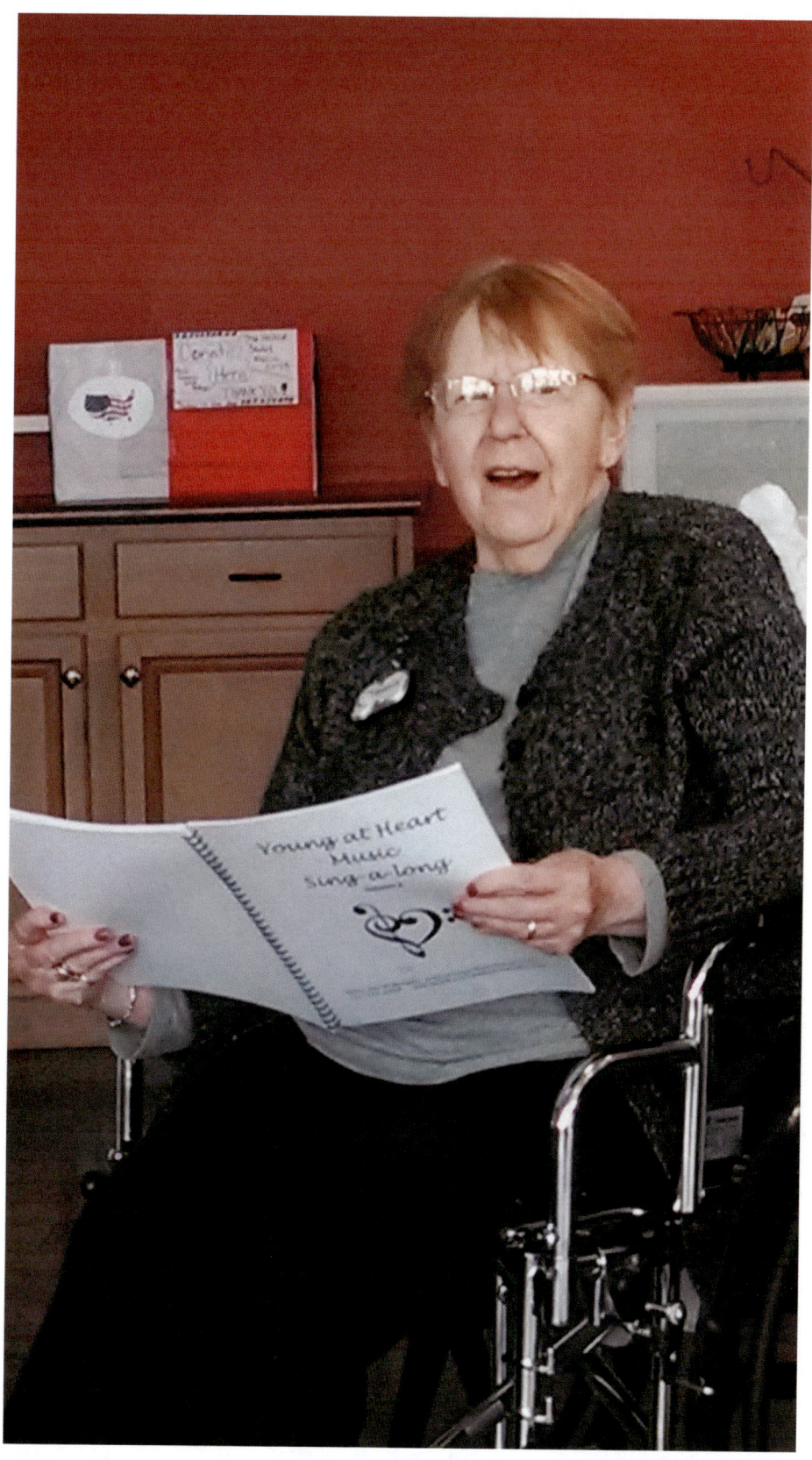

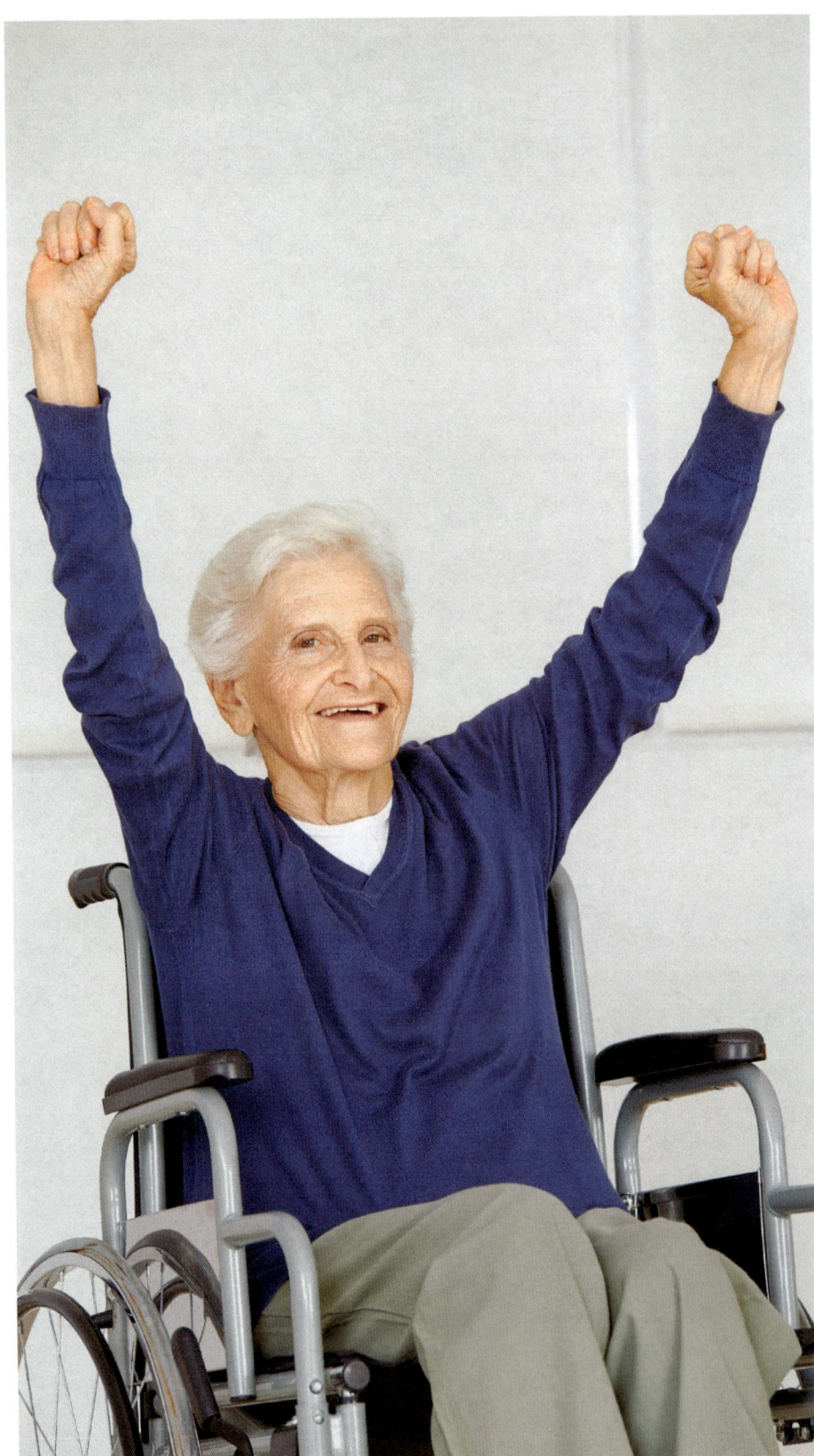

Chapter 8

Connecting Music to the GEMS™ Stages of Dementia

Introduction

The narratives and Music Moments in this section are here to help you gain a deeper understanding of characteristics associated with each GEM stage. This understanding, along with the guided questions, will help you plan for how to individualize and best use music on a daily basis. Keep in mind that the progression of dementia rarely follows a straight line. You may have experience with only one or with many of the GEMS over the course of your care giving.

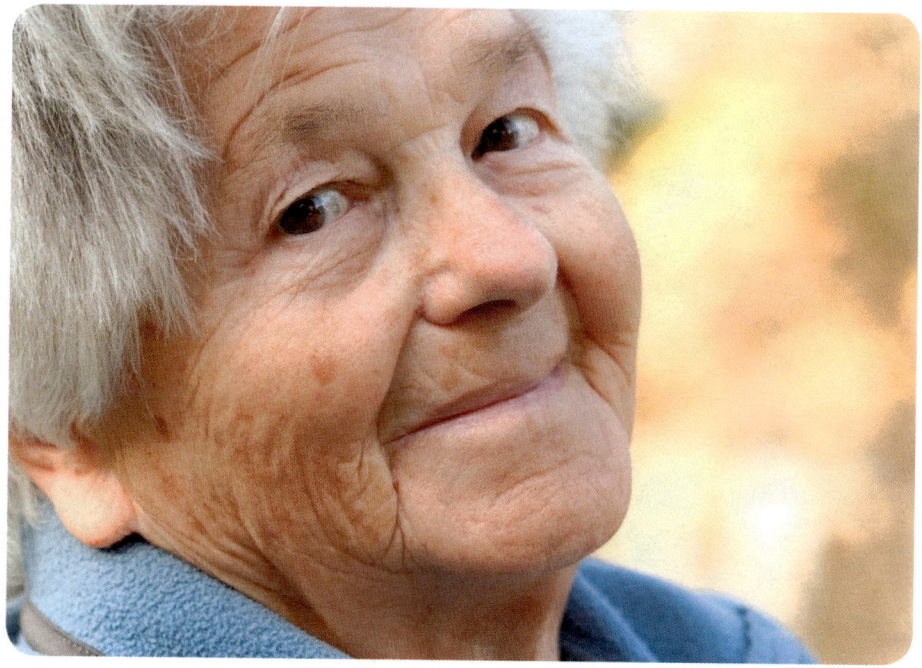

Diamonds - Clear and Sharp - Routines and Rituals Rule

Diamonds like routine and they can tell you what type of music they like. They may even be harshly critical if you play music they don't like. They need emotional connection to the people in their lives—and music provides it! Diamonds may like to sing the same songs over and over. It may be difficult for them to learn new songs. They are able to engage in music-related games, including "finish the line," "name that tune," and music trivia challenges. Diamonds will enjoy discussing music and memories related to songs.

A "Diamond" Music Moment with Mary Sue

The first time I met Elizabeth she was grumpy, a perpetual scowl painted on her face. But after our first time singing together, she told me a story.

Elizabeth said, "My dad died when I was young and my mom was left with just us three girls. Every night we would sing. We were so poor we didn't have enough money for a piano. But we sang and we sang and it helped get us through that time and lifted our spirits."

Elizabeth comes to singing almost every time now—and she tells me this story almost every time, too. I never mind hearing it again.

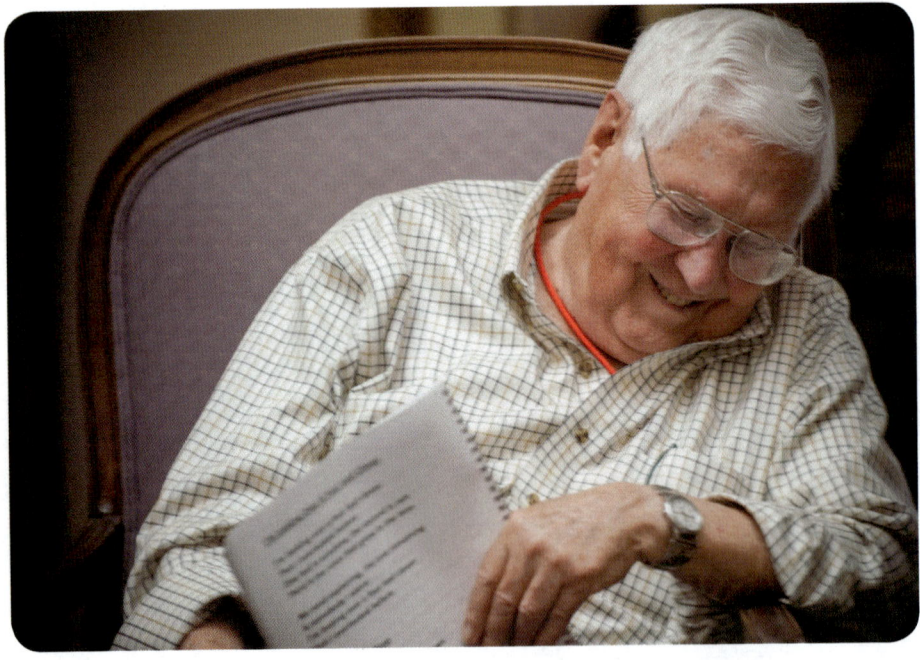

Think about the person you are caring for:
What do you see that makes you think they are a **Diamond**?

Describe a situation where using music will help either you or the person you care for or both:

Think about what your goal is for that situation:
Here are some ideas: Soothe, Energize, Connect, Entertain, Move from point A to point B, Distract and Redirect, other?

Think about how you will use music:
What song(s) and/or movement might you use? (Refer to the songs in this guide for examples.)

Think about when and where you will try this:
Get specific about the time, place, and location.

Emeralds - Green and On the Go with a Purpose - Naturally Flawed

Language becomes more difficult for Emeralds, who often fear being perceived as incompetent. Singing familiar songs is a great way for them to feel competent and successful. Dancing and marching help their need to be "on the go." Because of the balance shifts required, dancing might help Emeralds maintain equilibrium and reduce the risk of falling. A specific song or piece of music may help remind them of transitions and personal care needed. Emeralds are still good at filling in the blank when given a song line or an expression, such as "shave and a haircut—two bits."

An "Emerald" Music Moment with Mary Sue

Right in front of me sits a woman with a round, soft face, tight curly hair, and the bluest eyes you can imagine. She is short and her feet barely touch the ground. She is wearing blue pants with tights underneath, and ankle socks that she frequently reaches down to pull up from her white tennis shoes.

She swings her feet and taps her toes to the music, often sitting on her hands like a small child might. She wears the biggest smile ever. When I arrive, she squeals, "I love you!" as she bounces up and down in her chair. Her voice is quivery, but she sings every song with gusto, often clapping along. Her delight in the music is contagious and spills over to those around her.

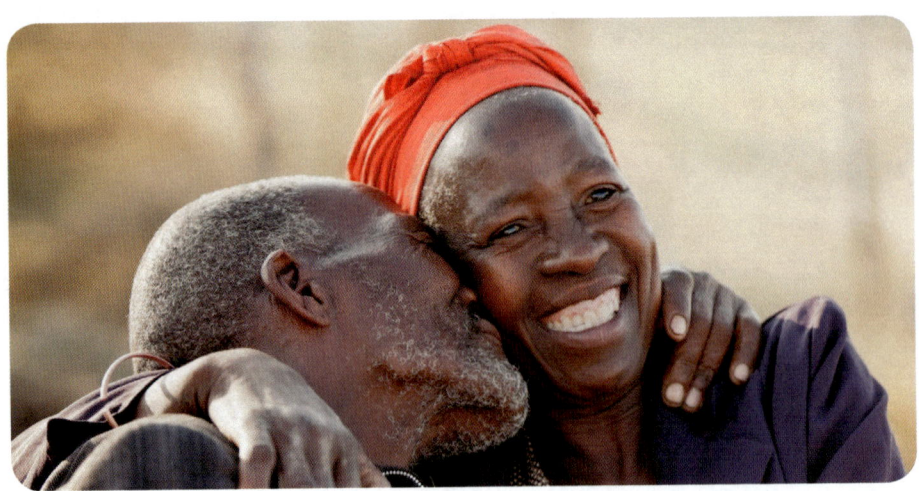

Think about the person you are caring for:
What do you see that makes you think they are an **Emerald**?

Describe a situation where using music will help either you or the person you care for or both:

Think about what your goal is for that situation:
Here are some ideas: Soothe, Energize, Connect, Entertain, Move from point A to point B, Distract and Redirect, other?

Think about how you will use music:
What song(s) and/or movement might you use? (Refer to the songs in this guide for examples.)

Think about when and where you will try this:
Get specific about the time, place, and location.

Ambers - Caught in a Moment of Time - Caution Required

Ambers will do what they like and won't do what they don't like. The best approach is to simply try songs and movement activities to discover their preferences. If they don't like something, come back later and try again. Music can be a way to engage, arouse, or calm an Amber who lives in the moment. Attention spans are shorter, so it's best to have music more often, though for shorter periods of time. Music will stimulate interest or memory in that moment. Since Ambers have little or no safety awareness, you should plan dance and movement space to insure safety. Ambers might prefer to watch or talk rather than participate. That's ok! Ambers are focused on sensation. If you encourage them to join you in a movement for a song, make sure to get permission to touch them.

An "Amber" Music Moment with Mary Sue

When I arrive at the adult day program, there are a dozen or so people sitting in a row of armchairs, waiting for me. They are singing "Let Me Call You Sweetheart." As I unpack my guitar, I introduce myself and join in. Several people compliment me on my shirt, which is pink and has shiny beads on it. We begin with "Hail, Hail the Gang's All Here." A few clap, and everyone sings and smiles. We are off to a good start.

A few numbers in, I launch into "Music! Music! Music!" Mary, who is sitting at the end with a walker in front of her, pushes to her feet and comes quickly to me. She grabs the neck of the guitar with one hand and my arm with the other and begins to dance. She moves in time to the music and leads me, stepping side to side. Then Mary begins to pull my arms back and forth, front to back. I have to stop playing the guitar, but I keep singing, and the group sings along, too. Everyone claps when the dance is finished. I hug and thank Mary. What a delight to see her move so spontaneously in time to the music!

Think about the person you are caring for:
What do you see that makes you think they are an **Amber**?

Describe a situation where using music will help either you or the person you care for or both:

Think about what your goal is for that situation:
Here are some ideas: Soothe, Energize, Connect, Entertain, Move from point A to point B, Distract and Redirect, other?

Think about how you will use music:
What song(s) and/or movement might you use? (Refer to the songs in this guide for examples.)

Think about when and where you will try this:
Get specific about the time, place, and location.

Rubies - Deep and Strong in Color - Others Stop Seeing What is Possible

Rubies benefit from slower rhythms, such as those of waltzes. They can copy large movements but will not easily understand instructions. Show them movement with big gestures and demonstrations. Rubies have trouble starting and stopping, so take time with transitions. Don't tug or pull or force them. Repetition is valuable for Rubies, so don't hesitate to repeat songs and use short, simple melodies. The goal is to engage! Rubies will enjoy rhythmic interactions, such as singing, humming, rocking, swaying, and dancing. Rubies may be able to dance better than they can walk, but they cannot back up. Be aware of this when you are dancing, and plan for safety.

A "Ruby" Music Moment with Mary Sue

Many older people don't smile much. Their faces may appear expressionless, and when you ask them to smile, it almost seems hard for them.

Helen's face is different. She has a look of expectancy, not quite a smile. During our music times she often pushes back and forth in her wheelchair in response to the rhythm of the music. Her favorite song is "Home on the Range." Sometimes when we sing it, she is able to mouth the words "home" and "range." Helen also likes "You Are My Sunshine." When I get to the end of a line in the song, she nods her head, and I nod back, letting her know we are singing together.

Helen doesn't talk much at all anymore. She needs help eating and I haven't seen her walk in a long time. What Helen *can* still do is nod her head and let you know that she is enjoying the music.

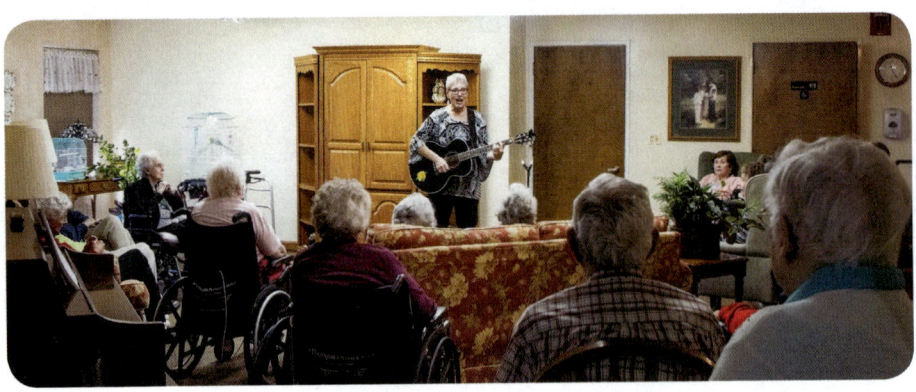

Think about the person you are caring for:
What do you see that makes you think they are a **Ruby**?

Describe a situation where using music will help either you or the person you care for or both:

Think about what your goal is for that situation:
Here are some ideas: Soothe, Energize, Connect, Entertain, Move from point A to point B, Distract and Redirect, other?

Think about how you will use music:
What song(s) and/or movement might you use? (Refer to the songs in this guide for examples.)

Think about when and where you will try this:
Get specific about the time, place, and location.

Pearls - Hidden Within a Shell - Beautiful Moments to Behold

Pearls are "hidden in a shell." You and the music can be the bridge that brings them out for short periods of time. Music will be experienced, but don't expect obvious visible response. It might be as slight as a smile, or a hand or foot moving. Be willing to accept and appreciate small signs of response. When providing music for Pearls, try to eliminate background noise so they aren't challenged or distracted. Offer it in a peaceful and private way, and see how open you can get the shell. Repetition is beneficial. Don't hesitate to sing the same song, gently, several times. Bring down the intensity by using quiet, slow rhythms to soothe. Pearls are beginning to have trouble swallowing; energetic music played a half hour before a meal may help get their lips moving and help them swallow.

A "Pearl" Music Moment with Mary Sue

Today I know the music session made Polly happy. Whenever I looked at her, she broke into a smile, nodded, and sometimes tried to sing along. There was something in her eyes that told me she was absolutely connected to me. I could hardly bring myself to look at anyone else because Polly's ability to communicate and connect is so limited. And because she was letting me know she was there. Today it was as if Polly had come to me from far, far away.

I don't cry often. The beauty of the connection today made me cry. It was one of the most profound experiences I have had with any of the people I sing with. What made today different?

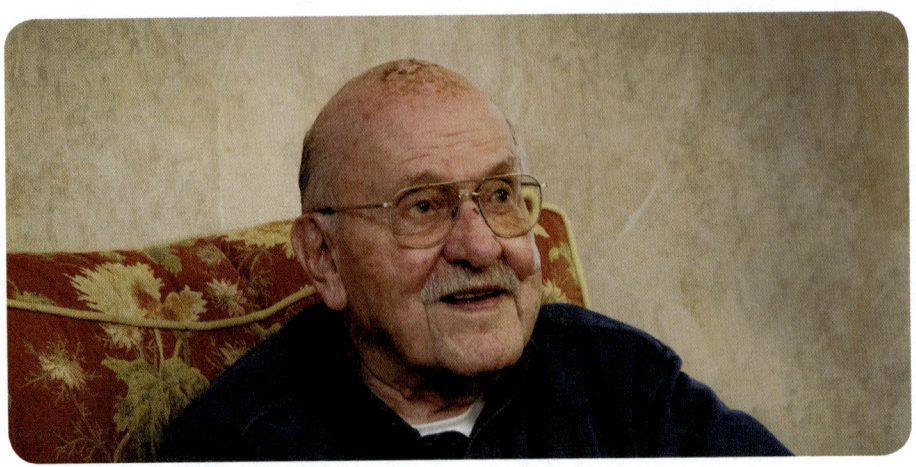

Think about the person you are caring for:
What do you see that makes you think they are a **Pearl**?

Describe a situation where using music will help either you or the person you care for or both:

Think about what your goal is for that situation:
Here are some ideas: Soothe, Energize, Connect, Entertain, Move from point A to point B, Distract and Redirect, other?

Think about how you will use music:
What song(s) and/or movement might you use? (Refer to the songs in this guide for examples.)

Think about when and where you will try this:
Get specific about the time, place, and location.

An Extra "Pearl" Music Moment with Mary Sue

Alec is a handsome man. He has Alzheimer's. He sits in a big, specialized wheelchair with a tray in front. Alec has difficulty hearing and most of the time he is asleep during music. He has never shown any response. Today he sat front and center, dozing as usual, while we sang Christmas songs, . But then I sang "Silent Night." Alec slowly drew his head up; I saw him struggle to open his eyes and gain focus. And then his face broke out into a beautiful smile as he looked right at me and said, "Wonderful, wonderful, wonderful."

I often use the word "awaken" when I describe what can happen with music. Today Alec's face showed the true meaning of the word. As he smiled through the song, I knelt down so I could look right at him and sing with him. When the song ended, I stroked his hand, leaned in, shared a smile, and thanked him.

We moved on to other songs. First up was "I've Been Working on the Railroad." Alec did not retreat! He stayed "in the music," dancing his hands on the tray in front of him, in time to the beat, beaming all the while. As the song went on, Alec reached his hands up to me. I took them, and together we swayed back and forth. He was connecting! I will never forget that smile or the magic of a single song.

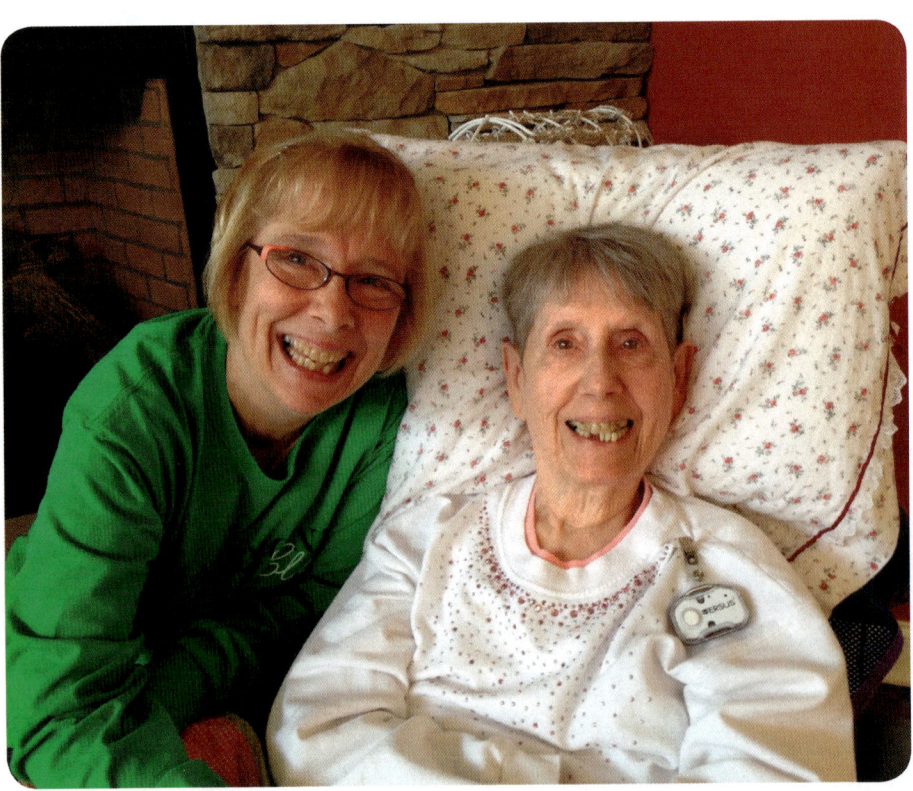

Your Notes

Online Resources

Singing Heart to Heart™, Mary Sue Wilkinson

www.SingingHeartToHeart.com

•••••••

Teepa Snow, Dementia Care Specialist, Positive Approach to Care™

www.teepasnow.com

•••••••

Pines Education Institute: Dementia Care Academy

www.dementiacareacademy.com

•••••••

Dementia Action Alliance

http://daanow.org/

•••••••

Alzheimer's Association

www.alz.org

•••••••

National Center for Creative Aging

www.creativeaging.org

•••••••

Music and Memory Organization

www.musicandmemory.org

•••••••

Alzheimer's and Dementia Weekly Newsletter

www.alzheimersweekly.com

•••••••

Daily Caring Newsletter and Resources

www.dailycaring.com

Bibliography

Aldridge, David A. *Music Therapy in Dementia Care.* London and Philadelphia: Jessica Kingsley Publishers, 2000.

An Evidence Review of the Impact of Participatory Arts on Older People. Edinburgh: Mental Health Foundation, 2011. http://www.mentalhealth.org.uk/publications/evidence-review-participatory-arts-older-people/

Clair, Alicia Ann and Jenny Memmott. *Therapeutic Uses of Music with Older Adults.* Silver Spring, MD: American Music Association, 2008.

Hamons, Meredith. *Musically Engaged Seniors: 40 Session Plans and Resources for a Vibrant Music Therapy Program.* Whelk and Waters Publishing, 2013.

Horn, Stacy. *Imperfect Harmony: Finding Happiness Singing with Others.* Chapel Hill, NC: Algonquin Books of Chapel Hill, 2013.

Levitan, Daniel J. *This is Your Brain on Music.* New York: Penguin Group, 2007.

———. *The World in Six Songs: How the Musical Brain Created Human Nature.* New York: Penguin Group, 2009.

Rhythmic Activities for Everyday Care. DVD and booklet. New York: Institute for Music and Neurological Function, 2007.

Rio, Robin. *Connecting Through Music with People with Dementia: A Guide for Caregivers.* London and Philadelphia: Jessica Kingsley Publishers, 2009.

Sacks, Oliver. *Musicophilia: Tales of Music and the Brain.* New York: Vintage Books, 2008.

Wan, Catherine Y., Theodor Ruuber, Anja Hohmann, Gottfried Schlaug. "The Therapeutic Effects of Singing in Neurological Disorders." *Music Perception*, Vol. 27, No. 4 (2010): 287-295.

Zeisel, John. *I'm Still Here: A New Philosophy of Alzheimer's Care.* New York and Toronto: Penguin Group, 2010.

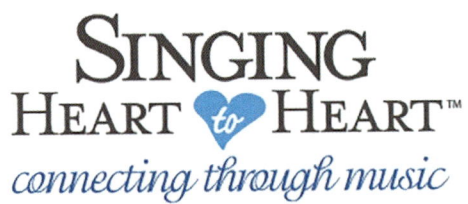

About Mary Sue Wilkinson and Singing Heart to Heart™

Mary Sue Wilkinson is the founder of **Singing Heart to Heart™** and the **Young at Heart Music Program**. She is a career educator and a professional musician. And she loves to sing!

Her flagship program, **Young at Heart Music**, is devoted to bringing the joy of music and singing to seniors with decades of life experience and memories tied to music.

Mary Sue is also a trainer and keynote speaker available to share her expertise about the power of music to awaken memories and bring joy. Her CD, *Songs You Know By Heart*, and her e-book, *Finding Memories through Music: A Family Interview*, as well as other resources are available on her website: **www.SingingHeartToHeart.com.**

Contact Mary Sue at: marysue@singinghearttoheart.com

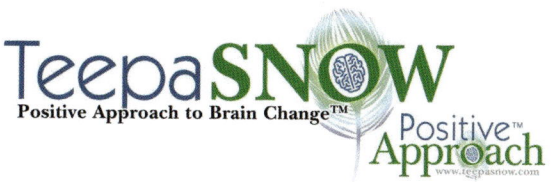

About Teepa Snow and Positive Approach to Care™

Today's Voice for Dementia, Teepa Snow is one of the world's leading advocates and educators for anyone living with dementia.

Teepa's philosophy is reflective of her education, work experience, medical research, and firsthand caregiving experiences. Her advocacy efforts led her to the development of the **GEMS™** dementia classification model and the **Positive Approach to Care™** training strategies.

An occupational therapist by trade, she graduated from Duke University and has an MS degree from the University of North Carolina at Chapel Hill. Teepa has impacted hundreds of organizations worldwide with her education, now reaching more than 30 countries.

Teepa's personal mission is to help others better understand how it feels to be living with dementia. She utilizes her gifts of role-play to demonstrate behavioral states and stages of dementia. This results in greater understanding for her audiences.

Her company, **Positive Approach to Care**, was founded in 2006 and offers person-centered training opportunities in the United States, Canada, Australia, and the UK. Training options include dementia certification programs for professionals and hands-on skill training for family caregivers, community groups, and health care organizations. For further details, access to educational video clips, training tools, and other resources, visit **www.teepasnow.com.**

Many thanks to:

Melissa Coolman, who is so much more than my assistant. Thank you for your keen eye, your expertise, your thoughtful insights, and problem-solving skills. But most of all, thank you for your friendship.

My son, Jesse Rose, my daughter-in-love, Karla Jay, and my dad, for asking me every week, "How's the book coming?" Your genuine interest, encouragement, and love mean the world to me.

Amber and Rick Buist, for believing in me early on and entrusting me to sing with your father, Dick Buist, as he lived with Alzheimer's.

Kim Spencer, caregiver extraordinaire, for your smiles and kind words that always lift me up, for embracing the power of music in your care giving, and for your thoughtful insights.

Karen Bell, activity director extraordinaire, for introducing me to the work of Teepa Snow. You bring music and happiness to everyone in your sphere.

Teepa Snow and her staff for working so hard every day to make the world a better place, not only for people living with dementia, but for their family members and care partners as well. Your work has changed my life and inspires me beyond measure. Thank you for contributing to my book and supporting my work and the role of music in dementia care.

Special thanks to Pauline Weaner, whose picture you see with me on the cover. Pauline is 94 years young and is not living with dementia but agreed to have her photo on the cover because she believes in the power of music.

This book contains many photos from my work in the Young at Heart Music Program in Traverse City, Michigan. While most all of the people in the photographs are not living with dementia, they nevertheless gave permission for me to use their photos which I greatly appreciate. Additional thanks to family members who gave permission for me to use photos of their loved ones who are living with dementia or who have passed away.

This book came to fruition with the collaboration of many talented professionals. Each one contributed their skills, insights, and assistance along with genuine interest and support for the project. Sincere thanks to Susan McConnell/McConnell Communications, Jill Tewsley/Author Services, George Foster/Foster Covers, and Heather Shaw and Doug Weaver/Mission Point Press.

And finally, my heartfelt gratitude to Polly and Ann Ballou, and for all the people who have allowed me to share their lives and connect with them through music and song.

Your Notes

Made in the USA
Charleston, SC
25 March 2016